Cover Image Credit/Copyright Attribution: IIIerlok_Xolms/Shutterstock

Gudmund Ågotnes

The Institutional Practice

ON NURSING HOMES AND HOSPITALIZATIONS

Contents

Preface

Why nursing homes and why hospitalizations? The simple answer is because they, when combined, are simultaneously important *and* intriguing. Hospitalizations *matter*, for better or worse, for those hospitalized and those not, for the hospitalizee and for the hospitalizer. At the same time, decisions on hospitalization are not easily understood; they relate to various, complex factors, often in ways that appear perplexing. As an academic point of interest, then, analyzing hospitalizations can be both challenging and worthwhile.

It is an aim to speak about and to the practitioner, and, simultaneously, to the social sciences. Those who, from this book, expect concise recommendations to be applied within a field of practice will be disappointed. Rather than creating or even recommending practices, I seek to understand them, or more precisely; understand from where they are generated. It is still a most profound wish (and hope) that such an approach will be of relevance and interest for the field of practice. While it is not a main objective to speak on behalf of the practitioners in nursing homes, I believe this book can be read as an implicit advocacy for them - by describing the difficulties and the uncertainty caring staff have to relate to, and by describing the perpetual ambiguity influencing their work.

I am grateful for the help and support from many friends and colleagues, too many for all to be mentioned. Professors Karin Anna Petersen and Frode Fadnes Jacobsen should receive the largest amount of gratitude (and blame for any shortcomings); always helpful and inspiring. A very special thanks should also be directed to Staf Callewaert for an early and profound interest in the project and to Knut Ågotnes for guidance and discussions towards the latter phases. I am also indebted to the research project «Re-Imagining Long-Term Residential Care: An International Study of Promising Practices», by primary investigator professor Pat Armstrong, for including me in their project, and for conversations and practical help within and outside «my» project.

I am forever indebted those who hosted me for shorter and longer periods during fieldwork and other forms of data collection: the municipality for facilitation, the administration in the nursing homes for opening their doors, and the caring staff for sharing, showing, including and forbearance. All have been generous, some for granting formal access, some for that and much more: fearlessly sharing without receiving.

And, of course, to *Team Slim*.

Abstract

The main objective of this book is to analyze how and why nursing homes vary in practices of hospitalization of elderly residents. This objective will be approached through an analysis of *how practice is generated, shared and implemented in nursing homes, therein variation of practice*. The two levels of analysis - that of regimes of practice and of the specific practices of hospitalization - will be approached alternately; each elevating the understanding of the other in a continuous interplay.

Research literature states that rates of hospitalizations vary considerably between nursing home institutions, also within smaller geographical areas. In this book, explanations, causes and connections of practice are sought after through the analysis of factors on an institutional and structural level, and can, as such, be regarded as a supplement to the existing «knowledge bank» primarily addressing patient characteristics in analyses of hospitalizations from nursing homes.

The study aims to demonstrate how decisions regarding hospitalizations are derived from an *institutional practice*: implicit, informal, but still shared, effective and adequate, through an adaptation of Pierre Bourdieu's theory of practice. I will argue that *the institutional practice* is developed and implemented locally, in many cases related to the unit rather than the institution, based on a fundamental and encompassing *uncertainty* to which nursing home staff must relate. It will be further argued that the fundamental uncertainty, relevant also for specific decisions on hospitalization, relates to *continuity* (of many facets), to a larger degree than other factors analyzed.

Fieldwork, in the form of participant observation, has been conducted at six nursing homes in Norway, and two nursing homes respectively in Canada, the United States, and United Kingdom. The primary methodological approach is supplemented with interviews and statistical data.

Introduction

Residents of nursing homes are frequently hospitalized. They are also hospitalized differently: nursing homes have different thresholds of when to hospitalize residents and when not to. Given the gravity of such decisions – hospitalization for the frail elderly nursing home resident can be confusing, difficult and even deadly – such a variation appears as confounding. *Why do nursing home institutions adopt and execute different practices regarding hospitalization of residents?*

The question constitutes the foundation of this book. However, discussions and analyses will also cover practices in general in nursing homes, because the one cannot be understood without the other. Practices of hospitalization are not, as will be demonstrated throughout this book, predetermined either by patient characteristics, institutional characteristics, or structural frameworks. Nursing homes do not hospitalize frequently or infrequently exclusively because they have a certain segment of residents, exclusively because they are small or large, or exclusively because of the presiding legislation. Rather, practices of hospitalization are generated by those who practice, and are bounded in space by being shared within a collective of agents. Nursing homes hospitalize frequently or infrequently because of the incorporated practices of the respective nursing home staff, in other words. As such, practices of hospitalization are also related to the overarching question of practice in general. It will be argued that *an institutional practice,* implicit, unofficial and local, but still shared and effective, is prevalent in nursing homes, formed from *a fundamental uncertainty* among caring staff and generating *varied practices* between nursing homes.

1.1. Objectives

1.1.1. Primary objectives

The aim of the book is to contribute to the realm of understanding and explanations, rather than to evaluate and recommend practices for nursing homes.

The aim is not to identify a correct set of practices, but rather to understand and describe how practice «works». As such, the analysis is *about* rather than *for* the field of practice (Petersen & Callewaert 2013). Similarly, the study is one *about variation*, rather than one attempting to remedy unwanted variation. Rather than having the assumption of variation as an inherent evil (as is found in a majority of the research literature on hospitalization from nursing homes, see Chapter 4), I will attempt to analyze and explain how and why variation can occur.

It will be argued that practices of hospitalization cannot be understood solely through an analysis of the inherent characteristics of the institutions in which they are performed. Nor can practices of hospitalization be understood solely based on the specific decision-making process; that is, in total isolation from their wider surroundings. Rather, practices of hospitalization relate to an encompassing and general set of «how things are done», which are identifiable and bounded in time and space; described in the analysis as *the institutional practice*. Within the sample of nursing homes, there are no typical nursing homes with high or low rates of hospitalization; they cannot be clustered into groups of «similar traits and characteristics». The formal characteristics of nursing homes and the conditions to which they relate, do not *determine* rates of hospitalization. As such, comparing «nursing homes with high rates» with «nursing homes with low rates» becomes a moot point. *The institutional practice* transcends formal qualities in the sense of being unique and local, but still shared and adequate.

1.1.2. The role of comparison and generalizations

The nursing homes within the sample should not be considered representative of nursing homes in general, not even of nursing homes in Norway. The nursing homes are, however, *relevant* for nursing homes in Norway and elsewhere. The nursing homes speak to and about other nursing homes as well as the idea of «the nursing home». As for Prieur's «*Mema's House*» (1993: 25), our houses are cultural expressions, not by being equal to other houses or by representing a synthesized version of their «culture», but by being a comment to the world outside. That which is created in our houses can speak of something larger than the defined events transpiring inside the houses. As such, «representativeness» and «generalizability» commonly adapted in research on hospitalizations from nursing homes, takes a different meaning here. Instead of searching for common denominators (in the form of institutional characteristics) in a large sample of institutions (and in the process, transforming specific nursing homes to representative averages) the practice at *some* nursing homes will be analyzed. These practices are performed differently, and therefore produce potentially different outcomes, including rates of hospitalizations, *but are still based on the same dynamics*. To simplify and to borrow from Goffman (1959): the play evolves differently each time, based on participants, setting and context, but the fundamental rules of the game remain the same. In this sense, a practice that has universal qualities and therefore is relevant for all nursing homes and perhaps for other institutional settings as well will be analyzed. The objective, then, is the understanding of *modus operandi* (the process of generation, including potentially changing structuring forces) rather than *opus operatum* (the result/outcome) of practices (Bourdieu 2012: 18-19).

The undertaking of identifying practices that can be labelled as «representative» is also problematic. I will argue that the ways of doing things in nursing homes – *the institutional practice* – are shared and spatially bound, and relate to the respective institutional conditions and a structuring framework in an individual and non-deterministic way. Such an understanding makes the very undertaking of generalization problematic, perhaps even misleading. There might not be an arch-model (in a Weberian sense) to be found for the nursing home; the researchers' construction of one can therefore be considered a misrepresentation of diversity.

Problematic aspects of generalization notwithstanding, hospitalizations still happen, with considerable consequences for those involved. The institutional or local development of practices is no less real, relevant and important, even though they do not mirror that of *other* nursing homes in form and content. As an academic point of focus, practices of hospitalizations are also extremely relevant as they, in addition to their intrinsic value, speak of practice in general: the practices of hospitalizations are based, as it will be argued, on the more generally applicable practical sense shared in respective nursing homes. This practical sense, then, can be studied, understood and analyzed *through* the analysis of the specific practice of hospitalizations, while an understanding of practices of hospitalizations, simultaneously, must rely on an understanding of the institutional practice. In this way, decisions about hospitalizations can speak about practice in nursing homes and the relationship between practice and conditions *in general*.

1.1.3. Structure of text and international relevance

There are far too many aspects of nursing home life relevant to the specific study of hospitalization and the more general study of practice, for all to be included in the present analysis. Some elements, therefore, have been left out, leaving us with aspects of nursing home life more directly connected to practices of hospitalization.

The book is divided into four overarching parts (totalling 10 chapters), comprising an introductory part and an analysis in three parts. The introductory part consists of an introductory chapter, background and context of the Norwegian health care system (Chapter 2) and a presentation of the sample of nursing homes, hereafter called «our sample» (Chapter 3). In part one of the analysis, the theoretical and empirical phenomenon of *hospitalizations from nursing homes* will be analyzed from the vantage point of research literature (Chapter 4), a discussion of how hospitalizations can relate to conditional influences (Chapter 5), and how hospitalization, as a term and as an empirical phenomenon, can be understood (Chapter 6). In part two of the analysis, the perspective will be focused on a general understanding of nursing homes, through a discussion of the overarching tensions prevalent in all nursing homes (Chapter 7), and an analysis of nursing home residents and staff from our sample, and the routines to which they adhere (Chapter 8). In the third and main part of the analysis, the two levels of analysis, that of hospitalization and of the nursing home, will be fused in an analysis of *variation of practice*, through a discussion of the institutional practice (Chapter 9). The concluding chapter, Chapter 10, will synthesize and elaborate on the previous chapters, by discussing how variation of practice and variation of hospitalization can be understood and explained.

The study is primarily directed towards nursing homes in Norway. As the dynamics at play have a general quality, as will be argued, the succeeding discussions will hopefully have resonance outside the sector in question as well as outside our small country.

1.2. Methodology and beyond

1.2.1. Techniques and technicalities

The primary sample of the study consists of six nursing homes located in a Norwegian municipality. Only nursing homes with exclusively long-term beds are included. Long-term bed institutions must all relate similarly to the inherent dilemmas of whether or not to hospitalize their residents from what is considered their «home», and they share many of the same organizational characteristics, to which we will return.

The nursing homes included are to be found at the top and the bottom of a table of hospitalization rates including all nursing homes in the municipality. Three nursing homes with high hospitalization rates, and three with low rates are included in the study. In the nursing home with the highest rate of hospitalization, residents were 4.9 times as likely to be hospitalized compared to the nursing homes with the lowest rate. Of the six nursing homes included, two were public, three private non-profit, and one private for-profit.

Shortly after the selection process, the first phase of the data collection - multi-site participant observation - was conducted in all six nursing homes, in one nursing home at a time, for a two-week period. The fieldwork for each nursing home lasted on average five days per week, close to a full working day each day. Each fieldwork session started out with semi-structured interviews with the administrator, followed by semi-structured interviews with one or two head nurses in the units. This was followed by a «tour» of the facility, used both as an opportunity to get to know the units, and for residents and staff to be introduced to me and the project, albeit briefly. Typically, this was all completed within the first day of the fieldwork, leaving the remaining days for observational studies. Following the main objectives of the project, it was important to get as close as possible to the actual interaction among staff, and between staff and residents, as early in the project as possible. Consequently, as much time as possible was spent in the nursing home units. This general approach seemed to work well, and was therefore repeated at all six institutions. A majority of time was spent in one unit, again based on the objective of getting an in-depth knowledge of everyday life, as opposed to a broader overview of the organization as a whole. At the starting phase of each period of fieldwork, it was important not to overwhelm staff and residents (and the researcher). An approach was adopted of easing staff and residents into the (prying) presence of the outsider, while increasing the time spent in the units throughout the two-week period. This seemed to be a reasonable strategy; the staff certainly seemed to be more comfortable as time passed, paying gradually less attention to the researcher. Towards the end of the first week and for the remainder of the stay, the researcher spent entire shifts in the units, alternating between day- and evening-shift, with the former predominating.

During this phase of fieldwork, the role of the researcher at the institutions was closer to that of an observer than that of the traditional anthropological participant observer. Several hours were spent each day in the units, often in one sitting, observing everyday life. More often than not, the researcher would be seated in one of the common areas, trying to come to grips with, while simultaneously not interfering with, the flow and routines of staff and residents. That being said, it would be naïve to think that the researcher does not influence the object or phenomenon of study. Both during these two weeks and in a later, longer period of fieldwork, the researcher was, in many ways, an anomaly at the nursing home, not just as a «researcher», but also as a male in a predominantly female work environment, who came from a non-nursing background. Conversely, being an outsider, and being viewed as such by the insiders, also had its advantages: basic and naïve questions about the everyday life in the nursing homes could be asked, and were answered without hesitation or (apparent) scepticism. Being the unskilled outsider, in other words, provided an entry point to a form of informal rapport between the researcher and the staff members.

This phase of research was by no means limited only to observing; staff and residents would contact the researcher for small and large matters, all day, every day, and increasingly throughout the two weeks. Initiating conversations with residents also became more «natural» after a while. It seemed strange, problematic even, not to talk to residents while sitting in «their» common rooms, especially since the busy schedule of the staff seemed to leave them incapable of spending «quality time» with residents. Most of the residents welcomed all forms of interaction, and seemed to be deprived of outsiders to talk to. The conversations with staff also increased gradually, perhaps because of the increased interaction with residents, perhaps because the staff became familiar with the strange outsider. As much time as possible was also spent in the nurses' station, during morning and afternoon report meetings and during lunch; the only occasions where most of the staff were gathered at the same time. The nurses' station was an important arena of study as the dynamics of interaction in many ways contrasted with that of the rest of the nursing home. Not only were residents (for the most part) excluded from this arena, but it was also rare to have more than two staff members gathered for more than a minute outside the nurses' station; the busy schedule of everyday work simply did not allow for it. The nurses' station also allowed for a glimpse into the more informal aspects of work in nursing homes, as staff members would talk more freely amongst themselves, and to me, before or after report meetings, or during short coffee breaks.

After the first phase of short-term fieldwork and a period of data analysis, one of the six institutions was chosen for long-term fieldwork. The site for the long-term fieldwork, called *Acre Woods*, was considered to be the best option of the six based on several considerations. Acre Woods is one of the larger nursing homes, allowing for a larger research population. Additionally, the units at Acre Woods are divided strictly from each other, allowing for the study of more closed off social arenas as well as a comparison perspective between units at the nursing home. Convenience was also a factor; Acre Woods is located such that more time could be spent there than at other nursing homes. Shortly after choosing the site and meeting with administrators at Acre Woods, the long-term fieldwork was started, lasting approximately seven months, including holidays. As much time as possible was spent at the nursing home during this period. Excluding holidays, fieldwork was conducted at Acre Woods every week, between two to six days a week. The length of stay would vary more than during the short-term fieldwork, in part due to other obligations, in part because at times certain strategic hours were chosen, rather than entire shifts. For most days, however, the equivalence of one shift would be spent in the nursing home. As for the short-term fieldwork, the overall approach was along the lines of «less is more», in the sense that one unit, rather than the entire nursing home was prioritized. A main unit, later referred to as *the unit*, was chosen and became a starting point for all of the fieldwork. Approximately 70 percent of the total time was spent in *the unit*. The rest of the time was spent in other units, primarily one, later referred to as *the other unit*, and common areas outside the unit.

As for the role and physical positioning of the researcher during fieldwork at Acre Woods, there are more similarities with than differences from the short-term fieldwork. The role as «the observer» was, however, not as strictly maintained as previously, and became less defined as time passed. The role was not intentionally discarded, but was gradually altered through the influence of others, staff and residents equally, as they wanted and expected more involvement, feedback, conversations and small-talk. Towards the end of the fieldwork, the researcher's involvement at the nursing home had changed to include doing smaller chores initiated by staff, residents, and gradually, by myself, such as fetching and reading newspapers, refilling coffee and accompanying a resident to the activity centre.

The physical positioning, movement and interaction during fieldwork at Acre Woods was also similar to that of former fieldwork, particularly regarding an emphasis on common rooms, the nurses' station and hallways. In short, the biggest difference between the two phases was the longevity of the second phase which facilitated understanding and analysis of how practice is generated in a unit, while building on experience from and knowledge of other units and nursing homes.

Observational studies in nursing homes were supplemented, primarily in parallel, with other forms of data collection. Data on the formal characteristics of residents transfers to the specialized health sector was collected for a six-month period at Acre Woods (see Chapter 3.4), completed by nursing home staff.

Data on overall staff characteristics was collected for all six nursing homes, including information about age, tenure, gender, number of staff positions (percentage) and types of positions (permanent/non-permanent staff), all measured against the different professional groups (registered nurses, assisting nurses, assistants). The data was gathered directly from the institutions, providing up-to-date overviews of current staff (see Chapter 3.3.2). Obtaining the data directly from the source was beneficial in the sense that the administration could help to clarify uncertainties when analyzing the data. The data was provided in anonymized form.

Data on residents' characteristics was collected from Acre Woods. While raw data on staff characteristics was gathered from the institutions' electronic personnel programs (albeit these differed from institution to institution), the same could not be done for residents; this would not be possible without getting access to personalized information. Instead, data was collected manually, primarily from the respective unit leaders (see Chapter 3.3.4). The specific categories used to synthetize resident characteristics in an anonymized form were copied from an earlier Norwegian research project (Slagsvold 1986), allowing also for a comparison of our nursing home population with that of a similarly sized population from the 1980s (see Chapter 8.2.1).

After this relatively long period of data collection, all data, field notes, preliminary interviews and register data, were systematized and analyzed. Based on this analysis, unstructured interviews were conducted at each site with two or three informants, either from middle- or from upper management. A total of 15 interviews were carried out at this stage, adding to the interviews of a more informal character done at the beginning of the preliminary fieldwork. Nursing home- and unit leadership were targeted for this part of the data collection, as the previous parts, especially the fieldwork, primarily dealt with staff working more directly with residents. The interviews, conducted in one setting each time and lasting from 25 to 120 minutes, were based on an informal interview guide, and conducted at the respective nursing homes during working hours.

Also in parallel with the data collection described above, the researcher participated in a large international research project addressing promising practices in long-term residential care in North-America and Europe, titled «Re-Imagining Long-term Residential Care: An International Study of Promising Practices» (http://reltc.apps01.yorku.ca/). Co-contributors to this international project conducted fieldwork at two nursing homes respectively in the United States, the United Kingdom, Canada and Norway. At each site, two institutions were visited for a period of one week in total. The nursing homes visited as part of the larger research project will be referred to in the analysis, primarily but not exclusively with the objective of achieving an international, comparative perspective to the Norwegian nursing homes.

In addition to what could be considered original data material, considerable emphasis and time was directed at the relatively extensive research literature covering the topic of «hospitalization/transfer from nursing homes» (see Chapter 4), before entering the field. This was an important and time-consuming exercise, in part because of the background of the researcher, in part because of the sheer size of the research literature on the topic. The information and knowledge gained from the literature review was used to prepare the researcher for potentially relevant factors influencing decisions on hospitalizations, as well as providing an overview of how the literature emphasized the significance of relevant conditions. This knowledge was used more as a guiding principle than to determine the gaze of the researcher. Still, it was beneficial to gain such knowledge, in the sense of preparing the researcher with a torch to search in the dark, rather than looking at the one area already brightly lit. An overview of the research literature also provided an insight into areas not extensively covered, in part explicitly pointed out in the literature, facilitating an analysis that can be viewed as supplementary to the existing knowledge bank.

1.2.2. Theory of methodology

Having Bourdieu's theoretical universe as a pragmatic orientation rather than a governing schematic, methodological considerations are also affected. For Bourdieu, techniques, methodology, epistemology, theory of science and «theory» in general are inexplicably linked and overlapping (see also Prieur 2002: 109). One should not treat each aspect as independent from the others, as is more often than not the case, a position that has implications for the presentation of a text and not only the analytical process. With Bourdieu, the methods (techniques) of the researcher relate to her position and positioning towards methodology and epistemology, again dependent on the theoretical position in which she is situated.

As such, *this* researcher was positioned and was influenced by a theoretical orientation before and during the process of data collection, and during the process of analysis, although differently during and between the respective stages. Even though such an orientation is not to be understood as encompassing all aspects of the research process, particularly with regards to the overall design and analytical process, some fundamental theoretical pre-orientations should be accounted for as they, in part, guided the researcher during data collection. Before arriving at how, technically, the researcher was guided, the epistemological framework from which the techniques are derived must be accounted for.

Placing himself between or beyond (depending on how one reads) the traditions of subjectivism and objectivism, Bourdieu points to epistemological shortcomings on each side. Objectivism and/or structuralism, sometimes also referred to as structural objectivism (Bourdieu & Wacquant 1992) as an epistemological position, leaves the researcher incapable of grasping the fluidity and complexity of social life:

> *«The chief danger of the objectivist point of view is that, lacking a principle of generation of those regularities, it tends to slip from model to reality – to reify the structures it constructs by treating them as autonomous entities endowed with the ability to «act» in the manner of historical agents. Incapable of grasping practice other than negatively, as the mere execution of the model built by the analyst, objectivism ends up projecting into the minds of agents a (scholastic) vision of their practice that, paradoxically, it could only uncover because it methodically set aside the experience agents have of it.»*
> (Ibid.: 8)

«The objectivist point of view» can be distorting and reductionist, by projecting a «scholastic» logic of automatism, when applied to the study of practice. That is not to say that Bourdieu treats structural influences as non-existent, or as overtly relativistic, as seen within epistemological traditions described as «subjectivistic»:

> «It is good to recall, against certain mechanistic visions of action, that social agents construct social reality, individually and also collectively, we must be careful not to forget, as the interactionists and the ethnomethodologists often do, that they have not constructed the categories they put to work in this work of construction.» (Ibid.: 10)

To simplify a complex and nuanced theoretical framework: Bourdieu's agent can be found caught somewhere between structure and agency, his actions neither pre-determined nor completely rational or conscious, neither completely mechanical nor instrumental. For our benefit and in this context, the methodological implications of such a position are vital. Given such a position, understanding *practice* implies more than the analysis of *presentations or verbalizations* of practice. While the agent has a form of «practical mastery», he does not master the principles that structure the situation he is in. Agents' accounts of practice, therefore, do not include all aspects of practice. Such a position should not, however, be taken as an advocacy of the senselessness of the agent: «*It is because agents never know completely what they are doing that what they do has more sense than they know*» (Bourdieu 1990: 69). As will be addressed (Chapter 10), the practical sense of the agent has an unmatched accuracy, but such an accuracy cannot be recreated in its explicit intent. From a methodological perspective, agents' accounts are not sufficient in understanding the complexity of social interaction: simply asking, for the researcher, does not suffice. Bourdieu's epistemological critique of relying too much on what is being said is also connected to the researcher´s *treatment* of what is being said. The researcher will, in relying on accounts, objectify practice and ascribe to it a «sensible logic»; a misrepresentation both of the practical sense of the agent and of the «logic of the practice» it represents. Rather, practice «*(…) has a logic which is not that of the logician. This has to be acknowledged in order to avoid asking of it more logic than it can give, thereby condemning oneself either to wring incoherencies out of it or to thrust a forced coherence upon it*» (Bourdieu 1990: 86). Returning to the methodological implications of such a position, Bourdieu argues that there are three aspects of agents' accounts that are problematic for the researcher (Bourdieu 2012: 18). *«A discourse of familiarity»* implies that the informant unintentionally tends to exclude central aspects that he takes for granted that the researcher will also take for granted. The discourse represents more or less internalized knowledge that remains unspoken. *«An outsider-oriented discourse»*, implies that the informant tends to generalize and simplify, in part to adapt what is said to the researcher. The informant assumes the scope (or lack thereof) of the researcher's knowledge. *«A semi-theoretical disposition»*, implies that the informant's statements are quasi-theoretical and artificially reflective in the sense that he would like to impress the researcher and demonstrate mastery of the field of knowledge. Combined, primary sources of «the social» are, for the researcher, *perceptions* of «the social», taking the form of misrepresentations given to the researcher.

Such a position has explicit implications for the form of and reliance on interviews, which it has been argued elswhere as the: *«(...) most likely to generate the «official» native accounts of which Bourdieu is so distrustful»* (Jenkins 1992: 54). However, this epistemological critique is not only directed at research relying on interviews, or on the informant. A common critique of the traditional, methodological approach of anthropology, of which will not be elaborated on in detail here[1], is that, in a process of familiarizing herself with the unfamiliar, the researcher relies too heavily on verbal communication, that is of normative statements of what should happen, rather than «what really goes on» (Bourdieu 1990, 2003, 2012).

The misrepresentation of the agent by the researcher not only arises from relying on native accounts, but also from a tendency or a desire by the researcher to create representations that follow the structure and system of rules *in appearance* (Bourdieu 2012). Rules and patterns must be understood not as equal to practice, but as: *«(...) preserved by the group memory* [and] *are themselves the product of a small batch of schemes enabling agents to generate an infinity of practices adapted to endlessly changing situations, without those schemes ever being constituted as explicit principles»* (Ibid.: 16). The rules presented by the researcher are not absolute principles, nor do they, strictly speaking, determine *or* adequately depict practice. Misrepresentation on the part of the

---

1   Primarily as we find Bourdieu's critique of the methodological approaches in anthropology (for example Bourdieu 1990: 42-51, first published in 1980) somewhat generalized and antiquated, particularly in his presentation of the anthropologist as «the outsider» in a foreign environment.

researcher can, to summarize a complex discussion spanning several of Bourdieu´s texts, be traced back to a tendency or a need (Bourdieu is not specific on this matter) by the researcher to emphasize that which is apparent and available to her primarily through communication with informants. This tendency is again connected to the researcher's gaze towards *opus operatum*; towards that which is regular (and can be presented as regulating) and can be presented (in writing by the researcher) in a theoretical-logical fashion (Bourdieu 2012). The presentations of practice take the form of being logical, coherent and intentional.

> *«Just as the teaching of tennis, the violin, chess, dancing, or boxing breaks down into individual positions, steps, or moves, practices which integrate all these artificially isolated elementary units of behavior into the unity of an organized activity, so the informant's discourse, in which he strives to give himself the appearances of symbolic mastery of his practice, tends to draw attention to the most remarkable «moves», i.e. those most esteemed or reprehended, in the different social games (…), rather than to the principle from which these moves and all equally possible moves can be generated and which, belonging to the universe of the undisputed, most often remain in their implicit state.»* (Ibid.: 18-19)

The subtlest of pitfalls for the researcher, describes Bourdieu, is that descriptions of such patterns of practice are based on a vocabulary of rules, describing a social practice that relates to other conditions than that which is governed by rules (Ibid.). Practice, rather, should by studied for what it is, and not what is said about it. Or, as Jenkins´ summarized Bourdieu´s epistemological critique: *«It is not possible to read other minds, but it may be possible to step into others' shoes»* (Jenkins 1992: 50). Bourdieu does not describe in detail how the researcher should proceed, at least not in a technical sense, but rather criticizes methodological dogmatism and textbooks on methods as techniques. In the closing chapter of *Weight of the World* (1999a), contrarily, a methodological framework of sorts is presented, more descriptively than elsewhere. This study relied more heavily on interviews than previous work, and might as such (although apparently contradictive) be useful in a discussion of reliance on accounts. The specific text (Bourdieu 1999a: 607-626) is also relevant outside the setting of interviews and outside the context of the specific study, primarily in discussions of representations of informants (which, given the previous discussions, also relates to representations of agents). At the center of the argument made is an encouragement addressed to the researcher of avoiding *symbolic violence* (the imposition of meaning presented and experienced as legitimate) in practice (that is, through the concrete situation of the interviews) and in representations (that is, the textual, analytical presentations of the interviews). But good intentions are not sufficient in doing so: the relationship between the researcher and the informant is structured in a way that reaches beyond the *purposes* of the researcher.

Bourdieu addresses these structural discrepancies, which must be understood actively and approached by the researcher as part of a practice that can be «*methodological and reflexive*» without being the direct application of a method (understood as a technique) (Ibid.). To achieve a form of non-violent communication, the researcher must address the relationship as it is; as inherently asymmetrical. She must attempt (an important element; one can never fully *do*) to understand the content of the distance between researcher and informant, and their respective understanding of the research object. By doing so, the researcher can reduce, but never fully remove, distortions (Ibid). The asymmetry and consequent distortions must be approached as being automatic; the researcher sets the rules usually without negotiation, while the asymmetry can be further accentuated by differences in capital, as evident, for instance, in use of language. By addressing issues of social proximity and familiarity between the two, symbolic violence can be somewhat reduced. It is, however, not simply a question of creating a «*natural discourse*», but also of a thorough scientific construction of a discourse (a demanding and often overlooked exercise, it is argued), for instance through elaborate preparations, repeated interviews and supplementary methodological approaches (Ibid.). Although «distance» between researcher and informant is problematic in several ways, the researcher should seek to understand the position from which the interviewee speaks. This is not, it is stressed, the equivalent of the phenomenological understanding of «*projecting oneself to the other*», but rather of providing a «*generic and genetic comprehension*» of whom the informants are, based on a theoretical *and* practical understanding of the social conditions to which they are connected (Ibid.). Such an approach implies a detailed and thorough understanding of the mechanisms that influence the categories in which informants are placed, rather than merely having sympathy for them.

The approach can still be *sympathetic*, I will argue, in the sense of allowing for a mediation of those who are usually silenced (in a positional and literal sense), not by paraphrasing their statements, but by analytically understanding and bringing together their position and positioning. Such is the approach; the understanding of the position, positioning and practice of *caring staff*, through an analysis of practice and the conditions in which it is situated. This approach can further be said to draw on Bourdieu's methodological considerations in the sense that it will be an aim to reduce the exertion of symbolic violence, by not relying exclusively on accounts and by the application of a multitude of cohesive methodological/analytical approaches. Through such an approach, representations of caring staff that can simultaneously substantiate their important contribution *and* convey something more than what is readily available will be aimed at.

1.2.3. Socio analysis: from where does the researcher speak?

While the latter sub-chapter is primarily concerned with what has been described as a first *epistemological break* (in short: from that of commonsensical understandings and official accounts, see also introduction to Chapter 7) (Bourdieu et. al. 1991, Bourdieu & Wacquant 1992), this sub-chapter will concern itself with a second epistemological break, that is the presuppositions of *«(…) the «objective» observer who, seeking to interpret practices, tends to bring into the object the principles of his relation to the object»* (Bourdieu 1990: 27). Implied in such a break is a rigorous self-examination of and by the researcher (see also Prieur 2002: 109-11). Such an exercise is, again, connected to methodological approaches, through what has been labelled «participant objectification» (Bourdieu 2003) (as opposed to participant observation), described as: *«(…) a full sociological objectivation of the object AND of the subject's relation to the object»* (Bourdieu & Wacquant 1992: 68).

For Bourdieu, participant objectivation, not to be confused with the anthropological practice of writing oneself into the text, is the most challenging of scientific exercises, as it implies a break from all that is taken for granted. While stated as challenging, such a position can also be met with a fundamental critique in my opinion: the sociologist is presented as the sole agent capable of transcending the structuring forces hidden to all.

Although such a critique may not be thoroughly addressed by Bourdieu, he does provide some more or less detailed accounts of the researcher's endeavors in achieving a second break. The second break implies an analytical step away from the practice of the researcher (Bourdieu et. al. 1991), for example observation; an objectivation of the practice of objectivation in other words, but she is entitled to do so only on condition that she submits all acts of self-examination to rigorous *scientific* examination (Bourdieu 2003: 291-92).

In doing so, in my opinion, the role of the researcher is not only scrutinized but also made relevant, perhaps to the degree of representing an elitist position, for which Bourdieu can be criticized. Implied in this reasoning, although fairly hidden, lies an «objective truth», that is; available and objective knowledge can be comprehended and conveyed (albeit not readily available) by the researcher (as opposed to the informant). As such, the researcher is empowered; she *can* speak about more than what is obviously available, about more than perceptions of practice; her voice is more *authoritarian* in Jenkins´ terms (1992) than that of the informant. Looking at this reasoning from another perspective, Bourdieu can be said to place the researcher and the informants on equal terms; the researcher shares the social mechanism of her research object, she is part of the same dynamic, influenced by and relating to her past and her surroundings, as her informants are. As such, Bourdieu's epistemological critique also conveys the universal qualities of his theoretical framework, while also implying that the researcher should be an active part of what is researched.

This researcher is a product of scientific positions, not only that of the theoretical and methodological framework, but also that of being an anthropologist. The technical/methodological approaches applied are primarily anthropological, as is the mode of textual presentation, particularly the appliance of qualitative, empirical data in the text. The researcher has also been allowed to gain influence from other perspectives and approaches, most notably from sociological and health/nursing sciences, as well as from anthropologists working in-between different disciplines and areas of interest.

I believe that the strength (and simultaneously perhaps also the weakness) of this project lies in its many mothers and the different environments it addresses. This study, a bastard of sorts, applies a mode of analysis of a social phenomenon typical for sociology, adopts a sociologically oriented theoretical framework, applies methodological approaches and textual presentation typical for social anthropology, while simultaneously addressing a field of science best labelled as «health» or «nursing science». As such, this project can be labelled ambitious, perhaps also as pretentious, but also, simplistic and uncomplicated in a fundamental sense: the object of study has been the governing factor, rather than scientific techniques or traditions.

1.3. Clarifications and operationalization

The design of the project excludes potentially interesting and relevant areas of interest. Some areas not covered were done so by choice, other perhaps more problematic deficiencies are involuntary. I hope that these limitations are amended by continuously reflecting over their significance.

1.3.1. Limitations

Although a significant period was spent at several nursing homes, the researcher did not observe as many concrete cases involving a hospitalized resident as perhaps one would expect. Hospitalizations did not occur on a daily or even weekly basis, and many occurred at times when the researcher was not present (at night-time, for instance). Several such incidents are still included, through retrospective discussions and presentations of them by those involved. For several of these incidents, the researcher was familiar with «the cases» (and caring staff was familiar with the researcher's interest in them) as the decisions had the form of ongoing deliberations spanning several days, rather than sudden and/or acute occurrences. However, the primary empirical attention has been directed towards *decisions and/or considerations* about hospitalization, rather than actual hospitalization; decisions and considerations that are frequent in nursing homes. Furthermore, the primary analytical emphasis has been directed at how decisions on hospitalization relates to practice in general, a relationship that is, in my opinion, omnipresent in our and other nursing homes.

A contextual attribute of great importance for the practice of hospitalization not thoroughly discussed, is the organization- and location of hospitals (alternatively emergency wards) in relation to nursing homes. As the study is situated in one municipality, where all nursing homes are within reasonably similar distance to local hospitals, this aspect will remain under-communicated. For nursing homes elsewhere, however, distance to hospitals might be of great significance, also regarding hospitalization (see for instance Vossius et al. 2013).

Distance to hospitals can be said to be particularly significant in Norway, when considering the general topography of the country and the variation in distances between nursing homes and hospitals in various regions. Nursing homes with large distances to hospitals must, out of necessity, be differently equipped than nursing homes in close proximity to hospitals, for instance. Alas, this point, although important for understanding variation across larger areas, does not explain differences *within* municipalities. This theme is in need of additional emphasis among research communities.

1.3.2. Notes about words

«Hospitalization» is a politicized term, often including, as we shall see in Chapter 4, negative connotations relating to overutilization. It does not completely fit our purposes as it, technically, excludes *transfers* to emergency departments (see Chapter 6). A minority of research literature has adopted the term «transfer» instead, which, most commonly, does not account for the difference between acute and non-acute transfers. I will use the term «hospitalization», in part because it is the most commonly adopted term, in part because it implies a level of gravity for those involved, primarily by excluding appointments and check-ups at hospitals.

The term *«resident»* is problematic as it downplays the multi-faceted and complex forms of difficulties for elderly people living in nursing homes; perhaps to the point of romanticizing. Nevertheless, the term will be used as the alternatives, «patient» and «elderly person», are equally inadequate and carry their own distorting connotations. In nursing homes, «patient» is often the preferred term, and will be quoted as such when used by nursing home staff.

The term *«care»* will be used, covering several aspects of nursing home life. The term will be used as it is in an emic sense, that is as it is used by nursing home staff, covering both the Norwegian «omsorg» (care as a general approach and/or a philosophy), and «pleie» and «stell» (the concrete actions performed by staff with residents). The term is inadequate in the sense that it includes multiple, sometimes even contradictory levels of meaning. «Care» can refer to an action as an object (the action of administering medicine for instance, included in the Norwegian «pleie»), and/or to the normative aspect of actions (that of providing something more profound than technical assistance, included in the Norwegian term «omsorg»), perhaps even contradicting one another.

Although not completely adequate to our purposes, a more precise and encompassing term(s) was not found.

The primary protagonists of this book will be labelled *«caring staff»*, translatable to the Norwegian «pleiere»: a construct on the part of the researcher, comprised of assistants, assisting nurses and registered nurses, and equivalents of each respective category. In research literature, «nurses» is sometimes adopted referring to equivalent groups (and might or might not include groups not technically «nurses», most notably assistants). The term «caring staff» is useful, in my opinion, as is signifies a distinct separation from those who do not provide direct care to residents: administration, kitchen-, maintenance-, and cleaning staff and (to some degree) physicians.

As already made clear, this study predominantly draws its data from two, related sources: fieldwork conducted at six nursing homes in a larger city in Norway and fieldwork conducted in eight institutions (six of which are outside Norway). The former will be considered primary, the latter supplementary. In the discussions of international or cross-jurisdictional relevance, the six nursing homes from Norway will be labelled «the national sample», the remaining nursing homes «the international sample». In other discussions, the label «our nursing homes» or «our sample» will refer to the primary institutions: six nursing homes located in a larger Norwegian municipality.

1.4. Meeting a resident; the curious case of Cate

One of the advantages of doing fieldwork for an extensive period of time at a nursing home is the possibility of observing the interaction between staff and residents over time, in different periods and stages of a resident's life at in the nursing homes, and, in some cases, from the very beginning of their stay.

Cate

Cate is, as all her co-residents, not capable of properly caring for herself. She had been living alone, taking care of herself, with no help except from close family members, before suffering from a stroke. The stroke left her incapable of walking and her speech was left severely slurred. Of all the residents in the unit, Cate struck me as the loneliest and as the one with the most desperate need for attention and affection. This was despite the fact that, as I later found out, a daughter visited her almost every day, visits which she seemed to treasure and enjoy.

Cate moved into the nursing home shortly after I started my extensive fieldwork in the unit. She moved in on a Friday afternoon during early winter. I first met her the following Monday. At the time, I did not know of her arrival, only that another resident had died shortly before, which always meant that another resident would be moving in shortly after. When attending the morning report meeting on Monday morning, Cate was pretty much the sole focus. The assisting unit leader was in charge and described how Cate's first days had been. Usually, a single resident did not get the sole attention of the morning report meeting, but it was deemed necessary on this occasion. Cate had, according to the assisting unit leader, been *uneasy* and *did not settle down*[2] for the entire weekend. *She´s very alert and present*, she continued, *but has some loss of speech and is confined to a wheelchair because of a stroke*. The assisting unit leader continued describing how Cate had been confused and scared, including at night. During the weekend, a caring staff member had to be with her at all times. The assisting unit leader concluded the meeting by telling all members to be extra attentive to Cate's needs, and that they somehow had to make her more comfortable in the nursing home.

During the week, I met, observed and talked to Cate every day. Before supper on Monday, she sat in the small common room together with the usual group. To my surprise, she was calm, smiling, and talked to several of the other residents, who, although having great difficulty in understanding her, tried their best to include her. Cate was, then and in general, extremely outgoing, always trying to make contact and smiling to everyone approaching her. On this particular day, and as usual, she was well dressed, wearing nice jewellery, and, even though having a somewhat untidy hairdo, presented herself as a «nice lady». She immediately took a liking to me, perhaps mainly because she felt lost and lonely and I could give her more attention than the caring staff could afford. She waved me in, smiling, giving the impression of having something urgent and important to convey, of which I did not understand much. All the same, she responded gladly when I simply smiled back or said *yes, that's right*.

The following day, Tuesday, Cate's behaviour was very different, and resembled the description of her by the assisting unit leader. Sitting in the same common room, with the same co-residents, at approximately the same time, she now cried and

---

2   A term difficult to translate from the Norwegian «å finne roen».

sobbed, trying to get the attention of everyone walking by. Now, she seemed to be seeking attention to comfort or help her, rather than simply someone to talk with. One of her neighbours addressed me: *Poor thing, she´s been like this all day. Nothing helps.* Cate fidgeted in her wheelchair, not finding a comfortable position. At one time, she let out a moan when shifting position, indicating that she was in pain. An assisting nurse came shortly thereafter. She told me that Cate had been uneasy all day, including the entire night, not getting any sleep at all. A night nurse had been with her all night. The only thing that seemed to help was to stroll her around the unit in her wheelchair, which the assisting nurse was about to do, while simultaneously seeing other residents in their rooms. For the remainder of the shift, an assisting nurse accompanied Cate at all times, or rather; Cate accompanied a nurse while the latter was doing other tasks.

The following day, Cate was better, but not completely. She alternated between short rests (finally caving in for lack of sleep, I thought) and being uneasy and restless. Her restlessness was not as distinct as the previous day, however, and talking to her seemed to calm her down. She did not need a member of the caring staff present at all times, but they often checked in on her.

The fourth day, Thursday, saw another change: for the entire day, she was all smiles, seeking contact with everyone around her, laughing when someone approached. She had a habit, exhibited that day, of grabbing your hand, grasping on to it and giving it gentle strokes, while at the same time keeping you close. Cate also had found her appetite again, which had been missing for the two previous days. During the afternoon report meeting an assisting nurse conveyed her thoughts, saying that Cate was much better, but that she did not understand if it was a question of adjusting to the nursing home, recently administered medication or a passing physical illness that had led to the change.

The following week, Cate's situation had changed yet again. For the first two days of the week, she was again very restless and uneasy. At the Monday morning report meeting, a registered nurse explained that Cate had *been up* during the entire weekend, including night-time, to the frustration of night-time staff. This state had continued throughout the day, and it seemed to be sustained. *It is imperative that someone is with her at all times. When she´s in this state it only takes a minute or two,* marked the end of the update on Cate. After the report meeting, I asked the registered nurse about what she had meant by the dangers of leaving Cate alone (at the time, relatively new to nursing homes, I took it to mean that Cate would get upset if left alone for too long). After some discussion, it became evident that the registered nurse was talking about the dangers of Cate falling out of her wheelchair when confused and restless. She had fallen four times (!) during the last couple of days, and had previously, before coming to the nursing home, had a fracture in the femoral neck.

For the next three days, someone was by Cate's side at all times. Usually it was a student (the nursing home had just received nursing students on internships in the nursing home from a university college), sometimes assisting nurses or assistants, sometimes me. For most of the time, she had to be walked around the unit; simply sitting and talking to her did not calm her for long. Therefore, and unlike any other residents, she attended all report meetings and other meetings in the office of the unit leader, always enjoying herself and, apparently, relishing the attention. As opposed to the previous week, the report meetings now revolved more around Cate's psychotropic medication, of which several had been tried out. The assisting unit leader and another registered nurse talked about the different kinds of medication, which they in turn had discussed with the physician, and debated their respective effects with the rest of the staff. The general consensus was that none of the psychotropic medication had the desired effect.

On the fourth day of the week, Cate's state changed abruptly once more. She appeared to be a totally different person than previously in that week, smiling, talking and being generally positive. In contrast to earlier, she did not doze off regularly or express feelings of pain. An assisting nurse told me Cate had slept through the entire night. Cate sat by herself most of this day, together with co-residents in the small common room, occasionally talking to other residents and staff who walked by, smiling to everyone who met her gaze.

Postscript:

About four weeks later, during a holiday period, Cate fell again, this time causing more damage than before. While attending an activity in the activity centre, without any staff from the unit present, she had fallen and broke a bone in her hip. Details around what happened were difficult to get hold of (I was not present), no one seemed to know exactly what had happened. Later, when talking to one of the activity personnel, it became clear that she had become restless during one of the activities and tried to stand up. The activity personnel further explained that Cate had stumbled on something on the floor and hit her hip on the floor when she fell. She made a point about the fact that no members of staff from the unit had accompanied Cate. Cate had been hospitalized immediately after the incident, and had returned to the unit shortly thereafter. Following the hospitalization, Cate was put on another, presumably stronger, scheme of psychotropic drugs, which had a marked and lasting effect on her: from this period and for the remaining six months of my fieldwork, Cate became calmer, had fewer changes in mood, and fewer «bad days». She did not fall again. However, Cate also became far more docile, sleepy and less enthusiastic. She seemed to me to be in a constant state of drowsiness, seldom showing her outgoing and enthusiastic features that both caring staff and residents appreciated.

Background and context

Contextual and structural features to which nursing homes relate do not determine practice at the nursing home, as will be argued. In general, to synthesize an argument discussed in more detail later, contextual and structural features can be viewed as a road map (Prieur & Sestoft 2006: 32-33); describing different and specific alternatives and trajectories. Neither the road one chooses, the direction one travels, nor how one travels – the practice – is given from constructing or reading the map. Still, context, background and structure matter, both for the agent (who must relate to them), for the institution (which *is* situated in Norway), and for the reader.

2.1. Norway in a nutshell

While empirical data and contextual features from Norway will be primary, discussions will also have relevance outside of Norway. The first part of this chapter, describing different contextual layers to which nursing homes relate, is primarily directed towards readers not overtly familiar with healthcare in Norway, giving brief, general summaries of the respective topics.

Norway, as a welfare state, offers what is defined as «universal benefits and services» to its inhabitants. Education, financial benefits and healthcare, should, according to this doctrine, be provided based on need rather than affluence or social status. Although the term «universal» might not be technically accurate in the sense of offering *equal* health care to *all* inhabitants, Norway does offer its inhabitants a comprehensive social and health security system compared to other countries. This security system includes what is widely considered affordable care for elderly people in need of social and/or medical care, the forms of which we will return to later. The healthcare system in Norway (and other Scandinavian countries) is generally described as being representative of the Nordic welfare system. The Nordic welfare system, although internally varied, has been described as a «social democratic» version of the welfare state, as opposed to «corporatist» and «liberal» models. The Nordic version differs from others most notably in its degree of promoting equality of access to services (Esping-Andersen 1990).

2.2. Nursing homes in Norway

Nursing homes have played a pivotal role in Norwegian eldercare for decades, and remain today an exceptionally important institution for the care of the elderly, even compared to other Scandinavian countries (Armstrong et al. 2009). Nursing homes in Norway, as in many other countries, provide a level of care somewhere between the specialized care sector – hospitals for instance – and home based care. In Norway, all nursing homes, private and public, are subject to national health legislation, in contrast to both Sweden and Denmark. Compared to other OECD countries, Norway is in the top echelon of expenditure on long-term care, both in absolute numbers and relative share of gross domestic product (OECD 2013). In other words, Norway has a high level of expenditure on care for the elderly measured against comparable countries, perhaps not only because it has revenues to spend, but also because care for the elderly is widely considered a public domain. Care for the elderly is part of the Norwegian, and to some extent Scandinavian, notion of the welfare state, and nursing homes can be said to be its most important part. The relative importance of nursing homes in Norway can be illustrated by the fact that 43.3 percent of all deaths occur in nursing home institutions (Krüger et al. 2011: 1)[1]. The particular topography and geography of Norway should also be taken into account when considering the importance of nursing homes. Norway is relatively sparsely populated over a large (relative to number of inhabitants) geographical area, has few large cities (most of which serve as regional centers), and has a topography and infrastructure making traveling long distances a challenge in many parts of the country. Many Norwegians therefore live far from hospitals and other parts of the specialized health service, both in distance and in travel time, giving the nursing homes a vital local function, as well as being a significant local employer.

In 2009 the total number of care recipients in long-term beds in Norwegian nursing homes was 34 800. This figure amounts to almost 1 percent of the total

---

1   Estimates from other countries are far lower: 24 percent for the United States and 18 percent for the United Kingdom (Phillips et al. 2006) in one study, and between 17 and 22 percent for the United States, in another (Bottrell et al. 2001).

population, far more than any comparable country[2]. Many elderly Norwegians live in nursing homes and the majority of these elderly also die in the nursing homes. Among residents occupying what is labelled a «long-term bed», it is estimated that 95 percent die while residing in the institutions (Husebø & Husebø 2005). The overall level of occupancy of Norwegian nursing homes, meanwhile, remains high, at approximately 98 percent[3] (www.ssb.no). The high coverage can be related to the relative (compared to number of elderly) decline of total nursing home beds (Chapter 2.2.3), and is of particular relevance for future discussions regarding who reside in nursing homes and how staff relate to them (Chapter 8). In total, care for the elderly in Norway is therefore not only a public domain, but has been and is closely connected to institutionalized care, most notably nursing homes.

While this emphasis on public care is and has been a national endeavor, the implementation of care for the elderly takes place at the local level. In Norway, primary health care is decentralized: the municipalities are responsible for providing care for the elderly, including nursing homes, assisted living and home based care, while the specialist health care sector, including hospitals, is governed by the national health directorate. The separation and cooperation between these levels of care has been the focus of much public and scientific debate, especially concerning the transitions between the levels of care.

Most nursing homes in Norway consist of both long-term beds and short-term beds (or alternatively rehabilitation beds). Some, a minority, have only long-term beds, while a few have short-term beds exclusively. Short-term beds are either located in a separate unit, or integrated in the long-term bed units, depending on the size of the nursing home. Usually the short-term beds are in a minority compared to long-term beds at an institution. In the municipality hosting this study, a significant minority of nursing homes are exclusively for long-term residents (including all nursing homes within our sample), while a very small minority are exclusively for short-term residents. The number of short-term beds, although a minority, has increased in recent times, perhaps as a consequence of a new health reform, the so-called Coordination Reform.

---

2   In 2012 a federal rapport estimated that approximately 0.43 percent of the total population resided in nursing homes in the United States. As opposed to the mentioned number for Norway, this estimate includes short-term beds (National Center for Health Statistics 2013)

3   Including older people's homes. Coverage, while high in total, varies somewhat between municipalities (www.ssb.no) (see also Chapter 2.2.4).

Nursing homes in Norway can be further divided into public, private non-profit and private for-profit. The division is similar to the organization of long-term residential care in the rest of Scandinavia and North America, while being distributed differently: there are more public and less for-profit nursing homes in Norway. The majority of nursing homes are public, quite a lot are private non-profit, and a few, mostly in the larger cities, are private for-profit.

Within the municipality included in this study, institutional size varies considerably, from that which can be considered small (even by Norwegian standards), with approximately 15 residents, to that which can be considered large by Norwegian standards, with well over 100 residents. The average size of nursing homes is over 50 beds. A small majority of nursing homes are public, many are private non-profit, while a few are private for-profit. Most of the nursing homes combine long- and short-term residents. As for Norway in general, the nursing homes that combine long- and short-term beds have more long- than short-term residents.

2.2.1. Financing

Recipients of care partly finance the primary healthcare sector through payment for services offered calculated in relation to individual income[4]. For nursing home residents, the individual payment is 85 percent of the pension, paid to the federal state. Although residents have to pay a portion of their pension, they will retain other assets, as opposed to the United States, for instance. Individual payment should in general not be higher than what is considered «affordable» (NOU 2004). The payment by nursing home residents should cover all care and support given at the institution, with minor exceptions, such as individually adjusted care aides (typically individualized care aides provided by occupational therapy services), and food and beverages not offered by the nursing homes, such as sweets and wine. The institutions do not, however, receive payment directly from their residents, but are financed by the municipalities based on number of residents (based on specific «rates» of short- and long-term beds, respectively). To simplify: elderly persons not in employment receive a pension from the federal

---

4   For all expenditure on public healthcare in Norway it is calculated that 85 percent is covered by the government, while 15 percent is covered by direct payments from the recipient (Stortingsmelding nr. 26 2015: 41).

government of which there is a minimal amount. Residents of nursing homes pay a part of this pension back to the federal government as payment for services offered. The municipalities receive their income from the federal government as block grant funding, while a portion is calculated based on taxes paid within the respective municipalities, which have relative autonomy over how much they chose to spend on care for the elderly. The nursing homes receive a fixed amount of revenue from the municipalities based on number of beds. The relative «income» for the nursing homes, that is to say the revenue per bed, should be the same, regardless of ownership, size and location.

The financing model results in two, perhaps paradoxical, traits of Norwegian nursing homes: *uniformity* and *autonomy*, traits to which we will return. The healthcare sector in general can be described as *uniform* in the sense that access is determined (or should be determined) solely based on necessity, that institutions receive a flat rate of reimbursement regardless of who applies, and that admissions criteria are similar for all nursing homes. The municipalities, meanwhile, have some *autonomy* in the sense that they can allocate the income from the federal government independently, for instance in how many nursing home beds they choose to have, how many assisted living facilities and so on. The municipalities can also choose to offer eldercare themselves or outsource to private foundations or companies. Nursing homes also have a level of autonomy in the sense that they decide for themselves how to spend the fixed amount of income from the municipalities, including how to organize the workforce. The relative autonomy of the nursing homes also relates to the lack of formal regulations and guidelines, to which we shall return.

2.2.2. Staff

Depending on the size of nursing homes, the total number of administrative staff will differ, as well as the types of administrative positions. While all nursing homes have a head administrator, often but not always a nurse, usually only larger nursing homes have one or several positions hierarchically placed between head administrator and unit nurse, typically called «head nurse» and/ or «head of development», filling the role of middle management. Similarly, only larger and medium sized nursing homes have specific positions for finance and other administrative tasks, while smaller nursing homes divide these tasks between head administrator and unit nurse.

The caring staff at Norwegian nursing homes generally consists of registered nurses with a minimum of three years university/university college education, assisting nurses[5] with two year secondary school education and assistants without what is considered by the nursing homes as relevant education. Approximately 30 percent of all caring positions (excluding administration, maintenance, cleaning and kitchen staff) in Norwegian nursing homes are held by registered nurses, 46 percent by assisting nurses, and 24 percent by «other» (Gautun & Hermansen 2011). In total, 76 percent of positions are held by what has been deemed «relevant education» – registered nurses and assisting nurses (Fjær & Vabø 2013). The total number of positions covered by trained professionals is high in Norway compared to most countries, especially for registered nurses (Harrington et al. 2012). In general, registered nurses are a large and important professional group in healthcare in Norway. The importance of registered nurses is evident both in the amount of positions and types of positions in Norwegian nursing homes, and in the size and political capital of the Norwegian Council of Nurses (totaling approximately 90 000 members). Registered nurses often hold the position of head administrator/director, and almost without exception, as middle management and /unit leader.

Physicians' services for residents of nursing homes fall under the jurisdiction of the institution (through the municipalities), rather than the respective residents. There is no national norm or regulation stipulating coverage of physicians (per resident or otherwise) in nursing homes. Instead, the institutions are, by law, obligated to offer physicians' services to its residents by having a physician «connected to the nursing home», in some form. This arrangement is contrasted to practices where residents' private physicians follow them into the nursing homes, as seen in many countries such as Denmark and Germany (Vossius et al. 2013), as well as a combination of the two arrangements. Consequently, physicians «connected» to nursing homes are either employed and work *for* the institution directly (typically for private institutions) or are general practitioners often required by the municipalities (for instance through operation agreements) to work in nursing homes or other institutions (typically for public *and* private institutions). Physicians who work for the nursing

---

5   A term combining the Norwegian professional titles of «hjelpepleier», «omsorgsarbeider» and «helsefagsarbeider», and equivalent or similar to professional titles elsewhere such as «licensed vocational nurse», «licensed practical nurse» and «auxiliary nurse».

homes, typically at larger nursing homes, tend to have larger positions than those employed through the municipalities as they are responsible for a larger group of patients, while not necessarily limited by other forms of employment. As such, some physicians employed directly by the nursing homes only work with nursing home residents. Physicians employed through the municipalities, typically general practitioners, tend to work part time at, relatively speaking, smaller nursing homes. One study found that about 50 percent of physicians' services are performed by physicians in permanent positions (employed by the nursing homes), 50 percent in part-time positions (employed through the municipalities) (Krüger et al. 2011). This does not, however, imply that one in two nursing homes employ their physicians independently[6]. In general, physicians' employment at and collaboration with nursing homes are organized at a municipal level. Consequently, *how* physicians are employed at the institutions, including how much time they spend there, varies greatly between municipalities. As will be discussed, such a variation can also be found *within* a municipality, leading also to varying physician-caring staff relationships.

While physicians are employed differently from nursing home to nursing home, the total coverage of physicians in nursing homes should also be noted. On average, there is one fulltime physician position per 127 nursing home beds in Norway, while for hospitals the coverage is one position per two hospital beds (Husebø & Husebø 2005). Another study from Norway points out that physicians were seldom available at the nursing home, in cases where people considered to be dying were hospitalized, arguing for better coverage by physicians in nursing homes (Hofacker et al. 2010).

Most nursing homes, usually depending on size, have staff for maintenance and cleaning separated from the caring staff. In general, larger nursing homes have a more distinct segregation of professional groups and a more distinct separation between professional and non-professional groups, compared to smaller ones. Most nursing homes will employ maintenance and cleaning staff themselves rather than outsourcing, although this trend is changing. When it comes to kitchen staff, generalizations are less adequate. Some larger nursing homes still have their own on-site kitchen, preparing warm meals for the

---

6   More than 50 percent of nursing homes will employ physicians through the municipalities in smaller positions, as larger nursing homes employ a larger relative bulk of physicians' services, thus increasing the overall percentage of physicians' services in full-time positions.

whole institution, while smaller nursing homes and increasingly larger ones as well, order meals from outside, to be heated on-site upon arrival. The former nursing homes will have separate kitchen staff, working exclusively with food preparation, while the latter will not, leaving the tasks of food preparation and presenting to caring staff.

2.2.3. Nursing homes compared to other levels of care

The 1950s saw the rise of both older people's homes[7] and nursing homes in Norway, replacing the traditional model of «care homes»[8] with little medical attention for residents (Hauge 2004). While older people's homes would provide a home-like environment for elderly people in need of limited care, the nursing homes would cater to the elderly in need of more extensive medical care, in a more medically oriented environment (Næss et al. 2013). This development was an integrated part of the post-war sentiment of larger public responsibility for those in need, and the gradual development of the welfare model. The rise of the nursing home in particular, should also be seen in the context of the general positivistic medical sentiment prevalent at the time, exemplified by the shift from addressing residents as «pensioners» to «patients», while simultaneously changing the outlook from institutions as places for retention of the elderly, to places of treatment (Hauge 2004). The nursing homes newly established in this period and throughout the 60s, bore the hallmarks of a concept of nursing homes as medically oriented facilities and were built accordingly, mimicking the architectural layout of hospital wings. Nursing homes became institutions where residents were considered patients in need of medical treatment, and thus an alternative to hospitals rather than a place of residency (Ibid., Næss et al. 2013). Consequently, nursing homes had an *intended* characteristic of temporality: «patients» were to receive treatment (and thus relieve the hospitals), before moving back home (Hauge 2004).

Such an intended function was both costly and not necessarily attuned to the characteristics of the nursing home residents, especially towards the end of what has been characterized as *«the period of treatment»* (1959-1980) (Ibid.). Gradually, nursing home residents became frailer during this period, in part as a

---

7   «Gamlehjem» or «aldershjem».
8   «Pleiehjem»

consequence of a gradual change towards more home-based services (Ibid.). Nursing homes had, once again, become institutions for retention. Consequently, during the following decades, starting from approximately 1980, several political and organizational changes were made. In 1988 the primary health services were decentralized, leaving nursing homes as the formal responsibility of the municipalities[9]. The municipalities, not being allocated specified government funding for nursing homes, dedicated resources towards home based care, further raising the criteria for admittance to nursing homes (Ibid.). Also during the 80s and well into the 90s, older people's homes were increasingly replaced by nursing homes. At the same time, the number of long-term beds as opposed to short-term beds increased in nursing homes, gradually making nursing homes the last place of residency for residents (Jacobsen 2005). In other words, more elderly people resided in nursing homes for longer periods of time. Municipal autonomy and responsibility regarding healthcare can also be seen as related to the political principle, prevalent throughout the 1980s, termed «care at the lowest, most effective level possible»[10], wherein it is considered beneficial for patients to be treated at the lowest level (in terms of generalized treatment being low and specialized treatment being high), geographically close to their residence. The development of nursing homes during this period, including both their inherent characteristics and their relation to other forms of care, can be said to both follow and oppose the principle of «care at the lowest, most effective level possible»: municipal responsibility is in line with the principle, while an increase of long-term beds can be seen as opposing it.

In parallel with the organizational changes, political discourses about nursing homes have changed since the 1980s; nursing homes are increasingly seen as a place for permanent residence, accentuating the need to be «home-like» in political documents. (Hauge 2004). Accordingly, what nursing homes should look like has also changed significantly during the last couple of decades. Units are supposed to be smaller, preferably between 8 and 15 people (Fjær & Vabø (2013), while all rooms should be single occupancies with en suite bathrooms (Ministry of Health and Care services (HOD) 1989). New nursing homes are

---

9   Relative municipal autonomy is deeply entrenched in the Norwegian political history. Although recent political changes might alter the organization of municipalities (towards larger), municipal autonomy is still presented at an ideal to strive for: «*The reasoning for municipal autonomy stems from the idea that freedom for local priorities will provide higher quality of services, more correct priorities and more efficient use of resources*». (Stortingsmelding nr. 26 2015)

10   Translated from «Lavest- effektive- omsorgsnivå», «LEON» for short (see also Jacobsen 2005).

built in accordance with this standard, while many older nursing homes have been refurbished to comply with it (Otnes 2015). The gradual change towards a «home-like» institution should not, however, be seen as omnipotent. Nursing homes are still institutions for treatment, while incorporating ideologies and the aesthetics of the home (Hauge 2004). The nursing home has evolved into an institution serving multiple demands, resulting in tensions of multiple dimensions (see Chapter 7).

In total, «institutional care» in Norway has in recent history been more or less synonymous with nursing home care. As we shall see, there is a gradual and increasing change away from this widespread notion. Somewhat parallel to but also following the change from older people's homes to nursing homes, Norway saw another shift: a great increase in assisted living facilities and home based services compared to nursing homes. Relative to the size of the elderly population and contrary to popular belief, the number of beds in nursing homes has decreased from 1989 to 2006 (Gautun & Hermansen 2011, Næss & Vabø 2012), especially towards the end of this period, while remaining stable in recent years (Otnes 2015). Compared to the size of population aged 80 and above, the number of beds in nursing homes in 2006 was 53 percent of that in 1980 (Gautun & Hermansen 2011). In the same time period, the use of home-based services increased, as did the number of assisted living facilities, a development that has continued in recent years (Otnes 2015). In summary, more elderly people today, and more frail elderly people, are cared for in their home or in assisted living facilities rather than in nursing home institutions, relatively speaking.

The difference between the number of potential care recipients and the number of available beds in nursing homes is especially evident in larger cities. Registered nurses working in municipal health- and care services state that long-term beds are not sufficiently available today, especially in larger cities (Gautun & Hermansen 2011). The drop in nursing home beds relative to the elderly population implies, as we shall return to, that the threshold of admittance to nursing homes has changed over time, changing also, perhaps, the features and functions of «the nursing home». Even so, it should not be forgotten that nursing homes remain an important institution today: the absolute number of beds remains stable, while total expenditure in the nursing home sector remains high in an international context (OECD 2013).

The emphasis on care at home or in assisted living facilities should be seen as a direct result of policy priorities, especially the «Action Plan for Eldercare»[11] implemented nationally in 1997 (Næss & Vabø 2012). The action plan, whose overall objective was to reorganize municipal healthcare, brought with it two major changes for eldercare: 1) the restructuring of nursing homes, by adding new facilities and refurbishing old ones towards single occupancies with en suite bathrooms, and; 2) an increase in the building and use of assisted living facilities, the number of which nearly doubled between 1994 and 2008 and saw with it a substantial increase in new positions within the sector (Stortingsmelding nr. 26 2015, Næss & Vabø 2012). The use of assisted living facilities, then, has replaced older people's homes and, to some extent, the nursing homes' traditional long-term beds[12]. In total, however, the number of beds (nursing homes and assisted living) has decreased in the last 20 years, relative to the number of elderly aged 80 years and above (Gautun & Hermansen 2011, Næss & Vabø 2012).

One can make the argument that these developments, the strong emphasis on medically oriented care in nursing homes, and the increase in home help care and assisted living, have contributed to a larger division of care for the elderly. There is a large gap in services offered between these alternatives, even though assisted living facilities (a category in itself composed of different variations and categories) can be seen as a form of buffer between services offered in nursing homes and home help care. The threshold for receiving a long-term bed in a nursing home is far higher than for receiving home help care. Partly related to this discrepancy, partly to deal with the organizational distance between the general and specialized care sector, 2012 saw the heavily debated Coordination Reform (Stortingsmelding no. 47 2009). A main objective of this reform was to coordinate the cooperation between the levels of care, particularly between the nursing homes and hospitals, by transferring responsibility to the municipalities (Næss et al. 2013). For this context, one of the more specific intended consequences of the reform is to give the municipalities' incentives to accommodate the transfer of patients ready to leave hospitals to nursing homes, by penalizing them financially if they do not, thus reducing potential

---

11   «Handlingsplan for eldreomsorgen» (Stortingsmelding nr. 50 1997).

12   The national average of the number of residents in institutional care has decreased by 0.4 percent from 2013 to 2014, and by 1.8 percent from 2010 to 2014 (www.ssb.no).

and costly «bed-blockers» at the hospitals. The municipalities are, as a consequence of the reform, obliged to provide what is considered adequate health- and care support for discharged patients within the same day of discharge from hospitals.

The development of assisted living facilities and home help care can be interpreted in different ways. It can be interpreted as a return to the principle of «care at the lowest, most effective level possible», as assisted living facilities can be said to imply less of a change to residents' lives than nursing homes. The development can also be seen as being connected to a devaluation of the importance of long-term institutional care, where «the home» is seen as the ideal form of care for the elderly as opposed to «the institution». Alternatively, assisting living facilities can be viewed as the «new form of nursing homes», as an alternative form of long-term residential care offering, in many cases, 24 hours of available care. It has also been argued that there might be financial incentives to prioritize assisted living as opposed to nursing homes for the municipalities, as a larger bulk of reimbursements (particularly payment of rent) is covered by the federal government (Næss et al. 2013).

2.2.4. Local variations

The organization of nursing homes in Norway varies between regions as well as between cities and rural areas, both in regards to coverage (number of beds relative to number of elderly in need of beds) and level of staffing (Gautun & Hermansen 2011, SINTEF 2009). As the municipalities provide care for the elderly, the variation is often local. The variation in coverage of beds and level of staffing is directly related to the level of municipal income: richer municipalities have a larger and better-developed municipal care sector. Smaller municipalities tend to have more resources per capita than larger, contributing to the gap in quality and coverage between larger cities and rural areas. Coverage of physicians (measured as physician minutes per resident, per week), for instance, varies considerably between municipalities; from below 11 minutes to above 30 minutes per resident (Gautun & Hermansen 2011: 174)[13]. As we shall see later, coverage of physicians in nursing homes also varies

---

13 The national average of physician hours per week per resident for nursing homes is stated to be 0.49 (2014) by Statistics Norway (www.ssb.no), a figure well above the cited study. Differences might be attributed to different criteria of measurement.

considerably *within* municipalities. Interestingly, the number of elderly people with a need for institutional care is relatively higher in areas with lower coverage, especially larger cities, further contributing to a gap between need and availability (Ibid.).

Municipal autonomy in organizing and prioritizing nursing home care also leads to local variation in ownership status. One municipality might have only public nursing homes, while the neighboring municipality, with a different politically based leadership, might have outsourced all nursing home care to a private for-profit company. While the latter is rare, it is not exceptional.

2.2.5. Guidelines, regulations and accountability

The regulatory framework for Norwegian nursing homes can be divided into three interconnected levels: national health legislation, supervision and auditing on a county level and inspections by the municipality. All nursing homes in Norway are subject to health legislation (as opposed to for instance Sweden, where they are part of social care), formally under to the domain of the Ministry of Health and Care Services. Still, as we shall see, the bulk of the regulatory framework for nursing homes is placed at a local level of governance, the municipalities.

Municipal autonomy in providing care for the elderly is reinforced by the lack of strict government laws, regulations and guidelines for nursing homes, especially concerning patterns and level of staffing, and organization of work. The main instruments of regulation for municipal elder care do not specify how services should be organized, for instance, but rather state that written procedures should be in place (Vabø et al. 2013). One of the national regulations specifically targeted at nursing homes, «*Regulations for nursing homes and facilities with 24 hour services*», states that nursing homes should have a physician, a registered nurse and an administrator «*connected*» to it, but do not specify in which form and to what degree (Ministry of Health and Care Services (HOD) 1989). When it comes to total level of staffing «connected to the nursing home», the regulation states: «*The number of personnel otherwise necessary to secure residents necessary care and support*[14]» (Ibid.). In contrast to regulations on staffing, regulations on residents' rights are more concise,

---

14   My translation from: «*Det antall personer for øvrig nødvendig for å sikre beoer nødvendig omsorg og bistand*».

although they do not cover all aspects of residents' lives in nursing homes, stating for instance that residents should have individual rooms with telephone and WC. Another regulation targeted at nursing homes - *«Regulations for quality in care services»* - is similarly formulated in general terms, stressing for instance the importance of covering residents' *«fundamental needs»*, *«respect and security»* and *«independence»* (Ministry of Health and Care services (HOD) 2003 [1997]). The regulation endorses systems of internal control in nursing homes, in the form of written procedures (Vabø et al. 2013). The latter regulation has been demonstrated to have not been explicitly implemented in nursing homes (Sandvoll 2013). In general, the regulations described have the characteristics of framework acts (Vabø et al. 2013), rather than specific procedures and practices.

Besides the requirement to have written procedures and to have a physician and registered nurse available at all times (but not necessarily on-site), guidelines for staffing can therefore be described as general. While nursing homes are obligated to have *«sufficient and professional staffing»* (Ibid.), they are themselves responsible for determining what is *«sufficient»* and *«professional»*. In comparison to many other countries, there are no formal staffing requirements in place, for instance number of registered nurses compared to number of residents (Harrington et al. 2012). Also the requirement to have a physician and registered nurse available is largely an institutional discretion. While doing fieldwork in nursing homes, it became evident that several nursing homes interpreted «available» as being «on call» rather than present at the institutions, thus saving considerable expenditure.

Focus on the specific phenomenon of hospitalization, or in more general terms the transfer of residents from nursing homes to other (predominantly within the specialized) levels of care, is for the most part absent from national legislation. National legislation does cover treatment considered «life-prolonging» however, stating that residents can refuse when capable of doing so. When not, next of kin are given the legal right to consent to what is *«in line with the patient's presumed or actual wish(es)»* (Dreyer et al. 2010). Family members of nursing home residents, then, can potentially be influential in decisions of hospitalizations, to which we will return. Based on national legislation, it falls to the respective municipalities to formulate and implement guidelines for medical decisions concerning end-of-life care. Such guidelines are present for hospitals, but seldom for nursing homes (Husebø & Husebø 2004).

Nursing homes are in many cases left with the independent responsibility of creating such guidelines for themselves (only 2 out of 20 nursing homes did, in the cited study, Ibid.), or leaving the matter to the local staff, altogether: *«the professional uncertainty principle»* to which we will return.

«The Norwegian Board of Health Supervision» is the nationally recognized office responsible for the supervision of nursing homes' adherence to national legislation. While being a national institution under «The Ministry of Health and Care Services» and responsible for the overall supervision of healthcare[15], the actual inspections and audits are undertaken at a county level. «The Norwegian Board of Health Supervision» is mandated supervisory responsibilities for each county respectively, including all their nursing homes, regardless of ownership status. In contrast to the municipal inspections, supervision by the office is typically connected to a specific theme, altering from year to year. Inspections and audits are seldom for the entire operation of a nursing home, nor is it for all nursing homes within a county. While some inspections are planned and announced by the central office, the respective county offices can also initiate inspections for a specific institution or a municipality, based on information received from workers, families, users and/or media.

Aside from potential inspections from «The Norwegian Board of Health Supervision», it falls on the municipalities to evaluate and regulate nursing homes. As such a responsibility is placed on the municipalities, local variations are also found in this area. Typically, nursing homes are measured on *procedures* rather than *outcomes* (does the nursing home have and implement routines for fire safety, for instance) (Vabø et al. 2013). Usually, the municipal requirement is to have a written procedure, rather than an evaluation of said procedure, in place.

Within our municipality, a designated political-administrative department is formally responsible for all nursing homes. Both public and private nursing homes operate with a large degree of autonomy. Private nursing homes are eligible for inspections and must report to the municipality, but to a lesser extent than for public nursing homes. Meanwhile, the day-to-day business of operating the nursing homes is solely up the institutions themselves, including public nursing homes. Municipal representatives inspect all nursing homes annually. These inspections are for the benefit of the municipality and are not shaped

---

15   In addition to child welfare and social care.

or controlled by the federal government, nor does the municipality report its findings to the federal government. Even though not in the form of a regulatory body, the municipality is still heavily involved in providing services for nursing homes, particularly public ones, especially regarding employment of physicians and provider agreements covering various forms of goods and services.

Within the municipality, all general practitioners are obliged, through an operations agreement, to perform a portion of their workload at a nursing home or equivalent institution[16]. The municipal department coordinates the workload of the general practitioners in the public (and some of the private) nursing homes within the municipality. All physicians in public nursing homes are employed through this arrangement. Private nursing homes, meanwhile, *can choose* to use physicians' services through the municipality, or not, as some do (see Chapter 3.3.3). Private nursing homes are autonomous not only in type of employment for physicians, but also size of positions, in relation to the national legislative formulation of *«operating responsibly»*. Consequently, private nursing homes can vary considerably both in type and size of employment. Public nursing homes in the municipality, meanwhile, are provided with a norm from the municipality. Additionally, the municipality provides all nursing homes with various forms of provider agreements regarding food and other goods. Public nursing homes are obliged to adhere to the provider agreements, while private nursing homes decide on an individual basis.

The respective nursing homes must also relate to and communicate with the municipality regarding the intake process for new residents, regardless of ownership status. The municipality has sovereign authority in distributing residents to nursing homes, usually, but not always, related to geographical proximity. While this structure is universal within the municipality, the actual relationship and collaboration between nursing homes and municipal representatives differ regarding the intake process of new residents (see Chapter 5.2.).

2.2.6. Residents

The development and organization of nursing homes, assisted living and home-based care is related to the characteristics of the care recipients, and,

---

16   Specified in the operation agreement as being «public work» of which nursing homes is one alternative. Income for «duty work» at nursing homes is based on a fixed amount, and is considered less than income from a private GP position (Stortingsmelding nr. 26 2015: 127).

at the same time, to how care recipients are viewed by policymakers. Relatively more recipients today receive care at home or in assisted living facilities than in nursing homes, while residents of nursing homes are reported to have increased need for extensive care (SSB 2010, Næss & Vabø 2012). «The nursing home resident of today», as described in Chapter 8, is widely considered, in popular opinion, policy documents and research, to be physically and cognitively frail. Residents of nursing homes are presented as having a higher level of acuity than before, higher than what is ideal (in relationship to what is offered of care and treatment), and, to some extent, higher than in other countries.

The development of the organization of care for the elderly, regardless of possible changes to the elderly population in general, has an effect on which segment of the elderly population resides in nursing homes. Municipalities, especially the largest, *do* have a relative high threshold of admittance to nursing homes; residents should be considered to have extensive needs for medical and psychosocial care if they are to be considered eligible for a nursing home bed. Many municipalities, again especially in the larger cities, also have long waiting lists for admittance to nursing homes; from residents living at home, in assisting living facilities and from hospitals. As such, the relative downsizing of nursing homes in favor of assisting living facilities seems to have altered the general level of acuity for nursing home residents, and has influenced waiting lists and waiting time for admittance to nursing homes.

The general perception of the frailty of nursing home residents is supported by recent, national research: 76 percent of all residents of nursing homes are considered to have *«significant need of care»* (SSB 2010), making them a group ill fitted for care at home or even through assisted living. A study found that residents hospitalized from nursing homes in a large city in Norway had an average of 3.4 diagnoses at admission, while the average morbidity rate in nursing homes was 62 percent (Graverholt et al. 2011). Another study found that 81 percent of residents of nursing homes had a form of dementia, while psychotropic medication was given to 75 percent of these (Selbæk et al. 2007).

The elderly population in the municipality included in this study resembles that of Norway in general. Both populations can, in an international context, be described as homogeneous with respect to wealth, social class and ethnicity. Still, being a larger municipality, there are areas within its limits generally more affluent than others. Compared to Norway in general[17], the municipality is more ethnically diverse. This diversity has not yet reached nursing homes in the form of residents (as opposed to caring staff), many of whom are cared for at home, or simply have not yet reached old age.

In general, for the municipality and for Norway in general, nursing homes are increasingly a home for the frailest, oldest and most dependent elderly. When an elderly person is admitted to a long-term nursing home in Norway today, the chances are that the said person is in need of frequent and diverse care, has some form of dementia[18] and suffers from comorbidity in some form. This development parallels that of Sweden (Harnett et al. 2012). The level of acuity for nursing home residents, and how nursing home residents are *viewed*, is related to certain characteristics of nursing homes today, most notably that of being *medicalized* (see Chapter 7.2.3) *institutions* (see Chapter 7.2.1), offering *professional care* (see Chapter 7.2.2.) for *dependent and frail elderly* (see Chapter 8.2.).

2.2.7. Summary

The nursing home, as an institution, holds a significant historic and sociocultural position in Norway. Partly based on Norway's particular geography and topography, the nursing home has a local and national importance, surpassing that of alternative institutions, also compared to other countries. Even so, the number of nursing home beds has been in decline, both in total and relative numbers, while home-based services and assisted living facilities are on the rise.

Perhaps paradoxically, nursing homes in Norway can be described as exhibiting features of both variation and uniformity. The form of governance (municipal autonomy), lack of specific national guidelines and regulations, as well as Norway's geography and topography, lead to variation, or perhaps more precisely *facilitate the possibility of variation*, an important point in the later analysis. Meanwhile, ownership (a great majority of nursing homes are public)

---

17   Compared to other European countries, Norway has a relatively small population of «immigrants», or people not born in the country: 13 percent, most of whom originate from other European countries and can be described as «work migrants» (Stortingsmelding nr. 26 2015: 18).

18   In the research literature, «dementia» and «Alzheimer's» are alternately used to refer to the same diagnosis or disease. I prefer to use «dementia», as the term also covers «vascular dementia» (or dementia developed post-stroke), not technically classified as «Alzheimer's». When referring to researchers' explicit reference to «Alzheimer's», the latter will be used.

and the financing model secure a significant element of uniformity even across large distances. The financing model, a typical example of the welfare state emphasis on universal access, also contributes to relatively homogeneous groups of residents at various nursing homes with one important common feature; one has to be in dire need of a nursing home bed to receive one.

2.3. Facts (and some thoughts) about hospitalization

Rates of hospitalization from nursing homes are considered high in Norway, an assumption confirmed by the few studies addressing the issue explicitly (Graverholt et al. 2011, Krüger et al. 2011, Vossius et al. 2011). While also being costly, high rates of hospitalization are considered to be problematic as many residents may not benefit from this. *Variation* of rates between institutions (Graverholt et al. 2013) and regions (Vossius et al. 2011) has also been pointed out, adding to a general concern. However, knowledge of the magnitude of and reasons behind rates of hospitalization (and variation thereof) is scarce, as all the cited studies point out, particularly regarding potentially significant factors on a «cultural» and/or institutional level.

Applying quantitative, retrospective designs, similar to the design opted for by a majority of the international research literature, relevant studies point to high rates of hospitalization from Norwegian nursing homes compared to similar international studies. Graverholt, addressing the occurrence of *«acute hospital admissions»* from nursing homes in Bergen (the second largest city in Norway) during 2007-2008, found an annual rate of hospitalization for all nursing homes in the municipality at 0.62 per person-year (et al. 2011). Krüger reported similar figures, 570 per 1000 nursing home beds per year (et al. 2011), in a study of hospital admissions from 32 nursing homes in Bergen over a 12-month period. Vossius, meanwhile, differentiates between referrals to hospitals from the municipal of Stavanger (Norway's fourth largest city) and surrounding municipalities, finding different overall rates: 0.38 and 0.60 referrals per person per year, respectively (et al. 2013)[19]. The cited studies, it should be noted, have somewhat different criteria of

---

19   All three studies retrieved their data from the records of ambulance services, from which, it is argued, *«close to 100 percent of admissions from nursing homes to the hospitals are made»* (Krüger et al. 2011: 2).

inclusion to the object of study: Graverholt by excluding admissions to emergency departments and non-acute admissions (et al. 2011); Krüger by excluding admissions to emergency departments, while including elective admissions (et al. 2011); Vossius by including referrals both to hospitals and to emergency departments (et al. 2013). Median stay at hospitals for those hospitalized was three days (Graverholt et al. 2011), while the hospital mortality rate was reported to be 16 percent (Ibid.) and 7.8 percent (Vossius et al. 2013). The most common diagnoses for hospitalization were similar among the studies: respiratory diseases, fall-related and circulatory diseases (Graverholt et al. 2011), infections, fractures, cardiovascular and gastro-related diagnoses (Krüger et al. 2011), and falls, infection and respiratory problems (Vossius et al. 2013).

While two of the studies do not offer explanations for the relative high rate of hospitalization, Graverholt suggests that it can be connected to the fundamental understanding of the function of nursing homes in Norway and which treatments they should offer (et al. 2011). Based on such an understanding, it is hypothesized, Norwegian nursing homes might be more inclined to hospitalize frail residents than in other countries, specifically for acute conditions and palliative treatment (Ibid.). Conversely, the study also points out that the oldest residents in nursing homes are less likely to be hospitalized than their younger co-residents, adding to a confounding area of research - to which we will return in Chapter 4.

Even more interesting in our context than the overall rates of hospitalization, is the variation in hospitalization rates between institutions and regions. Institutional rates of hospitalization from within the same municipality have been shown to vary considerably: from 0.16 to 1.49 hospitalizations per person per year on average (Graverholt et al. 2013), a variation higher than comparable international studies (see Chapter 4). Rate variation between urban centers (the municipality of Stavanger) and rural areas (surrounding municipalities) has also been shown, averaging 0.38 and 0.60 referrals per person per year, respectively (Vossius et al. 2013). The difference in institutional rates of hospitalization is, it is argued, exceptional, considering the relatively small geographical area and assumed heterogeneity of the patient population (Graverholt et al. 2013). It is further argued that admission criteria, funding of services and physician time are «*fixed factors*», making the variation particularly conspicuous (Ibid.).

As for the overall rates, explanations for variation are not considered to be within the scope of the cited studies, although they do offer some suggestions. Vossius «*(…) assume that the reasons are complex*» and that «*(…) internal factors like staffing of the nursing homes and the attitude towards hospital referrals might contribute*» (et al.: 371). Graverholt, meanwhile, states that differences in «*professional cultures and organizational factors*», not included in their study, might be significant in explaining the perplexing variation (Graverholt et al. 2013).

How «attitudes» and «professional cultures» can influence decisions of hospitalization and thus explain potential variation of practices of hospitalization, will be addressed in the analysis. In doing so, the existing body of literature on the topic will be supplemented. The analysis of «professional culture» and «attitudes» will be added to by means of analyses of modes of employment for physicians, coverage of the different professional groups and significance of families of residents, among other potentially relevant factors. These two levels of analysis - one relatively exact and measurable, one complex and immaterial – will be fused together by treating the former not simply with regards to their formal qualities, but also how such qualities relate to «culture» and «attitude». Physician hours per resident will be analyzed in terms of implications for collaboration between physician and caring staff, for instance. The analysis of variation of hospitalization, I will argue, presupposes such a complex approach.

The nursing homes

For the sake of anonymization, our six nursing homes will not be presented in detail. Some information, which either could be identifying or is not considered crucial, will be left out, while still preserving the most important traits of the nursing homes. Some minor details about institutions and residents will also be altered throughout the discussion, to limit the possibility of recognizing individuals and/or institutions. As briefly mentioned in Chapter 1, the six nursing homes from the national sample are considered primary, and will be emphasized here, while the international sample will be referred to sporadically.

3.1. *Our* nursing homes

Acre Woods. The site for the extensive fieldwork, Acre Woods, a private, non-profit institution, is the largest nursing home in the sample. Acre Woods will be presented thoroughly throughout the book. A particular unit at Acre Woods can be considered primary, called «the unit» or «the main unit», in the following, contrasted by another unit at Acre Woods, called «the other unit».

Durmstrang. Durmstrang, a small nursing home, is the only private, for-profit nursing home from our sample. Certain aspects of Durmstrang will be presented and discussed in detail, particularly regarding employment of and collaboration with physicians and resident demography.

Galactic Manor. Galactic Manor, a small nursing home, is a private non-profit institution. The nursing home will be discussed in detail regarding staffing levels, physical layout and differences between units.

Emerald Gardens. Emerald Gardens, also a small, private non-profit nursing home, will be referred to particularly regarding acuity of residents, architectural layout and division of units.

Cloud House. Cloud House is a small, public nursing home, discussed in detail regarding physical layout, atmosphere and division of units.

Coruscant. Coruscant, a medium-sized public nursing home referred to sporadically, regarding composition of residents.

3.2. A day at a nursing home

While the typical characteristics of a nursing home can be explained easily in general terms, getting an impression of how everyday life in a nursing home unfolds can be more challenging, especially for the uninitiated. The typical events of a day at Acre Woods can therefore provide some insights into life in nursing homes. The excerpt is a synthesis of several days, highlighting typical occurrences, while noting daily variations when relevant.

Introduction:

Setting: *The unit* at Acre Woods. Number of staff on each shift varies, especially on dayshift. While the number of nurses and assistants is supposed to be constant (approximately 1 caring staff per 3.5 residents), the actual number depends on short- and long term sickness absence, maternity- and other forms of leave, and whether or not students are present. Actual coverage also depends on whether the unit leader and assistant leader participate in the direct care of residents (something they do at irregular intervals, and usually before 9.00), which again depends on the aforementioned factors. One alternating staff member is on «kitchen duty» throughout the entire shift, meaning that he or she will spend the entirety of the shift preparing food in the unit kitchen (supper is cooked in the larger kitchen serving the whole house) and cleaning up after meals. Cleaning staff are employed at the institution rather than the units, and are therefore not delegated to any specific unit, as opposed to caring staff. Cleaning staff are therefore not thought of as working *in* the unit. The unit leader and the assistant unit leader work day-shifts exclusively. The unit leader primarily performs administrative tasks, while the assistant unit leader divides her time between tasks relating to residents, primarily dealing with medication, and administrative tasks (planning the daily operations, for instance). Aside from the leaders, there are anywhere from five to eight caring staff members on a day-shift, including registered nurses, assisting nurses and assistants.

The daily routine:

The day-shift starts at 7.15 when the first batch of the day-shift arrive (others start later at different times) and overlaps with the night-shift until 7.30. Most of the day-shift start at 7.30 and go directly to a report meeting with a registered or assisting nurse who was present at the report meeting with the night staff. From 7.45 until approximately 9 all nurses and assistants are busy with morning routines in the residents' rooms. A few residents have already been attended to by the night staff, and wait in their rooms before «being taken out» by the morning staff. Usually they have to wait until the morning staff have seen to the rest of the residents. The majority of residents will be attended to by the morning staff.

The rhythm of events is predictable: unless there has been a special event during night-time or early morning, the same residents will be attended to at the same time, in the same sequence, every day. To organize the exact sequence of morning care, the staff is divided into two groups, each responsible for half of the residents. Some residents, a minority, need two staff members present during morning care, while others, also a minority, only need help with parts of morning care, most likely dressing and parts of the care connected to personal hygiene, and are self-sufficient when it comes other parts, such as going to the toilet. A few residents, typically two or three, will not be given their morning care at this time, as they have expressed the view, verbally or otherwise, that they want to stay in bed longer. All caring staff are busy inside the rooms of the residents at this time. When staff have finished the morning care for a resident, the resident is helped (a great majority of residents need some form of help moving to and from their rooms) to get to the large common area, where breakfast is served later, or to one of the smaller common areas. Other residents, meanwhile, will remain in their rooms until breakfast is served there. The same residents will eat either in the common areas or in their rooms, every day. A majority of the residents will eat breakfast in the large common area, and will be seated there while waiting for other residents or breakfast to be served. The common areas are gradually filled until 9.00. Depending on how fast the caring staff complete the morning care routines (depending on level of *actual* coverage), some of the caring staff might have five or ten minutes to spare to help with the preparation of breakfast before 9.00, mostly consisting of setting the table and preparing slices of bread. The designated kitchen staff will not be able to prepare everything themselves, and will need help at some point to be ready by 9.00.

During this period, and usually starting some time before, a nurse, usually the assistant unit leader, will administer the morning medicine. In addition to the registered nurses, several of the assisting nurses have taken the «medical course» making them eligible for administering medicine. This is a time consuming process, as it has to follow the correct procedures of checking medical journals and charts, and because a large majority of residents receive some form of medication. In the period shortly before breakfast, until halfway through breakfast, all caring staff are busy delivering medicine, preparing and serving breakfast, helping residents to and from the common areas and helping residents eat. Only three or four residents (a distinct minority) can make their own way to the common area, and can leave on their own. The rest need help, either to be transported to and from the common room, or to be fed. As mentioned, this is a hectic period for the staff; they will not have time for anything else, besides these necessary tasks. As time is of the essence, staff must change swiftly from one task to the next, and will have few opportunities to talk to residents aside from giving short comments. Towards the end of breakfast, things start to calm down. Some of the staff will find time to eat or drink a cup of coffee, or to sit and talk to residents for a short period. Residents in need of help, to get to the toilet or back to the rooms for instance, will more often than not cut these moments short. Meanwhile, breakfast is being cleaned up by caring and kitchen staff. About half of the residents who attend breakfast will stay behind either in the main common rooms, or in one of the smaller ones.

Immediately after breakfast, the caring staff gather in the nurses' station for reporting and further planning of the day. Most of the staff will be able to attend from the beginning, while some will arrive during the meeting or miss it altogether, either because of not finishing their respective tasks, or by an unforeseen task. If the unit leader or the assistant unit leader is attending (usually one, seldom both), one of these will take the lead. Depending on who's attending, who's leading the meeting and the general mood of the day, the meeting will proceed and focus on the remaining caring responsibilities and the organization of these responsibilities. Some days this is done swiftly and the topic often drifts to other, less serious matters. Most days, however, the staff only have time for the absolute necessities. If many experienced caring staff members are present, the morning rituals of the caring procedures are done more swiftly. Less time is also needed for planning and delegating if many experienced nurses are present; they know what to do and do not need to be told or to discuss amongst themselves. More often than not, a significant portion of the morning care will still remain at this point, consisting of residents who have not yet risen from bed, showering, or tasks connected to treatment of sudden illnesses, for instance. In addition, appointments for hairdressing and foot therapy are made most days. Caring staff have to prioritize accompanying residents to these appointments, as they are time specific. The appointments need to be addressed in detail at the report meeting, not only for the sake of the staff, but also to make sure that the residents are able to attend, which for various reasons usually connected to their physical wellbeing, is not always the case. The activities of the day, organized and taking place in the large common room of the nursing home, will also be discussed, specifically with regards to who is eligible for the respective activities, and which caring staff member should attend. The latter will depend on the needs of the respective residents as well as the availability of staff.

The meetings are informal in form; everyone is allowed to speak their minds, if not expected to. However, a select few usually have the center of attention, either by raising points or objecting to suggestions from the leaders. Should the planning not take the allotted time, the remaining minutes are used for a highly appreciated coffee break and small talk. Usually, there is no time.

From 10.15 until 11.30 three separate events occur at the same time: the remainder of morning care is finished, fruit is served, and the activity center is opened. The remainder of the morning care is the most time- and resource-consuming for the staff. Most of the caring staff will be busy with morning care until lunch, tending to residents who are bedridden, or have chosen to stay in bed late. Other residents will need to be helped when going to the toilet or to be accompanied to the hairdresser. At 10.30 fruit is served. Every resident will get a plate of fruit and a glass of lemonade. The designated kitchen staff will prepare the fruit, while some of the caring staff will help serve and help some of the residents to eat. The activity department, serving the entire nursing home, will arrange some sort of activity for the residents every working day. The activities will occur somewhere between 10.30 and 12.30, but not for the entire time. On average two residents from the unit will participate. Caring staff seldom have to stay by the resident's side during the entire activity. Sometimes it is necessary to accompany a resident, especially if the resident is thought to be «restless». If caring staff have to accompany a resident, the remaining caring staff will have difficulty in getting the remaining work finished in time. The original plan, devised at the morning meeting, will often not be fulfilled as intended; sometimes because the residents do not want to attend, but most often because staff get derailed by other tasks.

From 11.30 until 12.30 the staff have their lunch break. They are meant to divide themselves in two groups, with half an hour each, but the hectic schedule seldom allows them to. Most days the caring staff will eat when they can, and when it is suitable for others, usually for less than 30 minutes. There is a canteen available for all nursing home staff, but it is almost never used by caring staff from the units. For the caring staff, eating in the canteen is impractical, both in regard to the general hectic schedule, and the potential occurrence of an unforeseen event, leaving them, on most days, in the unit for the entirety of their shift.

Right after their lunch, caring staff start the preparations for dinner. Dinner is served around 13.00. Before this time, the frantic pace in the unit settles down remarkably. Morning care is now finished and most of the residents are resting or sleeping. The designated kitchen staff get help from several others in setting the table and rearranging the dining area. Other caring staff will finish whatever work is left over, work that is not top priority but still needs to be completed: changing beds, sorting clothes and making sure the different remedies and equipment are in place. Others will gradually get residents ready for supper; always in the same order, and always seated at the same place. As for other meals, residents are «made ready» for dinner well in advance, giving the caring staff the opportunity to get through all their designated tasks. When dinner is served, most of the caring staff will sit beside residents in need of various forms of assistance while eating. After dinner, many residents are accompanied back to their respective rooms, one by one. Some stay behind in the common rooms. Like breakfast, most residents will eat dinner in the common rooms, while a minority will be served in their rooms.

After dinner, the unit once again settles into a calmer pace. Most of the residents are sleeping, either in their rooms or in the large common room. A gradual shift of staff occurs between 14.00 and 15.00. Because of the extremely intricate shift plans, the respective shifts (day, evening and night) start and end at different times. Some will end their day-shift already at 14.00, while others will remain until 15.00 and will be able to attend the report meeting with the evening-shift, most of whom start at 14.00. The report meeting is between 14.00 and 14.30. Important messages concerning specific residents are the main topic of the meetings and will take most of the time. Compared to the day-shift, evening-shift staff do not spend much time on overall planning of the shift, primarily because they know that they have to be flexible regarding which tasks to do at what time, as there are relatively few staff members in relation to number of residents. There will always be enough tasks to fulfil, but it is hard to know which ones will be the most pressing.

The evening-shifts are extremely hectic from beginning to end. This seems to be connected to levels of staffing: usually (not taking into account sick leave and unexpected events) there is one caring staff member for approximately five residents, including the designated kitchen staff. The latter will alternate between kitchen duties and caring tasks more frequently than during the day-shift, as there are fewer tasks in the kitchen and more pressing demands relating to resident care. Still, when meals are prepared, each of the remaining caring staff members have to attend to more residents, making for a busy time and few opportunities to do anything other than what is absolutely needed. As opposed to the day-shift, there are few other staff in the unit at this time (physicians, maintenance staff, activity personnel and unit leaders). At all times there is one registered nurse on evening-shift serving the entire nursing home, hereafter called «the on-duty nurse», available for questions from and advice for the staff in the unit.

After the report meeting, there will usually be tasks to be performed consecutively during the entire shift. Coffee is served immediately after the meeting, usually with biscuits. At this time, more residents than before will remain in their rooms. The caring staff, therefore, constantly move between rooms, the kitchen and the common rooms. After coffee, the caring staff immediately start to administer medicine, together with other minor tasks that need to be addressed: cleaning, helping residents with their toilet visits, helping residents to and from their rooms, preparing for evening meals, and preparing for the bed routines.

The one activity that dominates the entire shift more than anything else is the bed routine. The bed routines are time consuming and therefore have to be done simultaneously with other tasks. Bed routines usually start at about 16.00. It is noticeable how similar the routines of helping residents to bed are from day to day. Regardless of who is on shift, the same residents are put to bed at the same time and in the same sequence, every day. As mentioned, this routine is done simultaneously with other tasks, partly because it lasts for a long time period. The routines of helping residents to bed are also connected to other tasks: when a resident has gone to bed, other tasks relating to the resident (such as helping with food, helping to and from the toilet, personal care et cetera) are also considered completed. Gradually then, from about 16.00, the total amount of tasks remaining for the evening-shift, diminishes. In this sense, and taking into account the hectic schedule of the evening-shift, the caring staff are strongly incentivized to attend to residents relatively early.

The residents can be divided into three groups in regards to how the staff relate to their bed routines: 1) residents who stay in the common area and are not capable of expressing the desire to go to bed; 2) residents who stay in their rooms, and; 3) residents who stay in the common room and who are able to express the desire to go to bed. The residents are almost without exception put to bed in the sequence of 1, 2 and 3. Within each of these categories we also find clear regularities in when residents are helped to bed. Category 1 consists of residents who stay in the large or the small common room during large parts of the day, have great physical caring needs, and/or advanced dementia and, consequently, difficulties in communicating. This category consists of 5-6 residents. Many of these residents are not capable of expressing their wishes concerning if and when they want to go to bed. Furthermore, regardless of being capable or not, residents are rarely asked whether or not they want to go to bed. Several of the residents have severely diminished physical capacity, and therefore are considered by staff to be «hard to care for» in the sense of being physically straining, prompting two or more staff members per resident. The need for two staff members per resident inclines staff to start the bed routines earlier for those particular residents.

After the bed routines are completed for category 1, the tasks connected to these residents will, as mentioned, be considered completed for the day. As residents are taken to bed, then, the total amount of tasks lessens, and time can be spent on other tasks, such as preparing evening meals, the bed routines for resident category 2, and other minor tasks postponed until now. During the first 5-6 hours of the evening-shift (from about 14.00 until approximately 19.30), there are few opportunities for staff to have a break or to spend «quality time» with residents. Given that six residents are in bed, it will now be 17.00 and the bed routines remain for a majority of residents. However, the remaining residents are easier to cope with than the residents already in bed. The remaining residents can be divided into residents who stay in their rooms, and residents who are still in the common rooms. The groups are evenly sized. Those who usually stay in their rooms, category 2, are a mixed group when it comes to physical and cognitive skills while those who usually stay in the common rooms, category 3, are relatively functional both physically and cognitively. From approximately 17.00 until 19.30 the staff tend to the bed routines for resident category 2. Some of these residents will also need two staff members present during the bed routines. During this period, especially towards the end, the evening meal is prepared and served, and the staff can take a short break to eat or to talk to residents

who are still awake. However, caring staff still have to be careful in timing their breaks, and can seldom take a break at the same time. As the evening unfolds, the tempo
of the units settles, since more residents are «finished» and the ratio of the number of
staff to residents gradually changes. Towards the end of this period, evening meals are
served to those who remain in the common rooms and to those who wish to have
evening meals served in their rooms.

The last category of residents, residents who have chosen to remain in one of the
common rooms, spend this relatively quiet time eating the evening meal, watching
television (which is on more or less all the time), and talking to staff who can finally
afford to spend time with the residents. Most of these residents will go to bed between
20.00 and 22.00, after expressing the desire to do so, as opposed to other residents.
Consequently, depending on the respective residents´ mood for the day, the exact
time when they go to bed will vary from day to day, again in opposition to other
residents, who do not have a say in the matter.

The evening-shift concludes with a report meeting between the evening- and night-
shift at 22.00. As with other report meetings, this is almost exclusively oral, even
though it is expected from the leadership that caring staff should read up on residents
in the electronic journal system. The night-shift is usually relatively uneventful, bar-
ring the occurrence of an unforeseen event. The night-shift staff follow a designated
pattern of doing rounds in the rooms, checking up on residents, providing medication and changing the sleeping position for those in need. Residents can, as often
happens, become restless during the night (see example from Cate, Chapter 1.4).
Usually the night-shift staff are prepared for such situations, as they are informed in
advance of potentially restless residents. The night-shift ends when the day-shift arrives at 7.15, and the report meeting is completed.

If an outsider were to describe the defining characteristics of the unit, the most
noteworthy would probably be the long corridor, the constant movement of the
staff, and the relatively clear distinction of resident groups (from both residents
and staff). The long corridor, identical to the corridors of the other units in this
nursing home, is important in the sense that it influences the level of mobility for
residents and staff alike. The corridor is long, reaching from one end of the unit to
the other, in one straight line. Consequently, staff and residents have to cover large
distances throughout the day. Staff constantly have to move from one part of the

unit to the other, taking up a fair amount of their precious time. Residents, most of whom are immobile to start with, have to cover a relatively large distance to get to their meals or to the toilet, especially if they are so unlucky as to have a room at the end of the corridor. The corridor also makes having an overview over the entire unit difficult. This physical layout is a contrast to most other nursing homes, where the corridors are shorter and often centered by a nurses' station or a large common room from where one can observe the respective corridors.

The constant movement of the staff is immediately noticeable in the unit. While this is a common observation at most if not all nursing homes, it is particularly apparent in this one. The constant movement of the staff is connected to the physical layout of the unit, but also, in my opinion, to something else. More so than at other nursing homes, and even in other units of this nursing home, caring staff are not supposed to have a slow pace, or to take breaks of any meaningful length, either for themselves or with residents (see also Jacobsen 2005). Caring staff are *supposed to be* busy, *supposed to* work hard, and *supposed to* preoccupy themselves. Caring staff who do not comply with this unwritten standard, particularly neophytes, are quickly sanctioned, directly or indirectly, by shrewd remarks such as *having a break again, are we?*

3.3. General characteristics of the nursing homes

Of the six institutions, two are located in the city center (Acre Woods being among those), while four are suburban. Two of the institutions are public, three are private non-profit (Acre Woods being among those), while one is private for-profit. The selection includes a disproportional number – four - of small nursing homes (between 20 and 40 beds). One of the included nursing homes is medium size and one is large (Acre Woods)[1]. Our nursing homes average 44 residents per institution, somewhat below the average of the municipality.

3.3.1. Units and common areas

All six nursing homes, regardless of total size, have some form of physical division of space, albeit in differing forms. The administration, for instance, is

---

1 Measuring the size of nursing homes is arbitrary, at least when comparing internationally. I therefore proclaim the right to categorize our nursing homes as «small, medium and large», based on a local scale, where small can be considered up to 40 residents, medium up to 70 residents, and large above 70 residents.

distinctively separated from the resident area, often by floor. The resident areas, the units, meanwhile, are separated from each other, in different forms. For all nursing homes except one, units are clearly separated by distinct entry points, usually a door with the name of the unit written on it, and by different forms of decoration or color schemes inside. At Uagodou, there are no barriers between the units; they are simply located in different corridors. Five of the nursing homes have relatively small units, with 8-12 residents, in line with recent policy trends. The last nursing home, Acre Woods, has larger units, with over 15 beds on average. Four of the nursing homes have separate units for residents who are considered to be a challenge to either control or care for, typically occupied by residents who are considered to have aggressive dementia. These units are defined as «dementia units», and have, in varying degrees, more security measures in place, especially locked entry points, and/or better staffing. All dementia units are separated from other units by floor.

Aside from administration and resident areas, all nursing homes have some sort of common area for visitors and/or residents. For three of the nursing homes these areas are larger and more commonly used than for the other three nursing homes. The common areas are located on the ground floor and serve both as activity centers for residents, who can attend organized activities with residents from other units during daytime, and as meeting points for when visitors come. For the other three nursing homes, the common areas are small, not commonly occupied by residents for longer periods of time (at least not in an organized form), but accessible for visitors and staff, sometimes accompanying a resident.

3.3.2. Staff

The caring staff constitutes, in several ways, the core of the nursing home. It is primarily to them that residents and visitors have to relate, while other professional groups, at least to some degree, are in place to better facilitate the relationship between caring staff and residents.

The caring staff at our nursing homes and, I would argue, nursing homes elsewhere in Norway, are relatively homogeneous regarding gender, age and social class, all themes we will return to. They are, however, increasingly heterogeneous regarding ethnicity. There is, in other words, increasing diversity of country of origin for caring staff, especially for nursing homes in the larger municipalities, such as ours. As our nursing homes do not vary substantially regarding cultural diversity of caring staff – a substantial number of assistants and assisting nurses at all nursing homes are foreign born, as are a minority of registered nurses at most nursing homes[2] - the topic will remain under-communicated. Caring staff of different national origin still constitute a large and important part of the work force in nursing homes[3]. A majority of caring staff of different national origin within our sample hail from Africa, South-East Asia or Eastern Europe. A disproportionately high number of these are assistants, some are assisting nurses[4], while a few (but increasingly more[5]) are registered nurses. *The reception* of caring staff with «other» national background than management and caring staff of Norwegian origin is, as experienced during fieldwork, extremely ambiguous, although generally reducible to a discourse of «the others» from the point of view of «the Norwegians». Some, both managers and caring staff, point to the absolute necessity of having a foreign work force, or, as one administrator put it, «*Without them we would be doomed!*» When it comes to abilities and approaches to work, most caring staff and management are clearly positioned; only a few are indifferent. Some point to the «softness» in physical care and the custom of taking care of one's elderly as important traits of the others, while some point to contradicting traits, claiming that the others are «too hard» and/or dismissive of residents' needs. A significant element of the discourse about the others is the language barrier between «them» and other staff members, and between «them» and residents:

We have large problems with language for the foreign speakers. As unit leader, I demand
that they are capable of speaking Norwegian to the residents, but still there are those

---

2   The data on staff characteristics provided by the nursing homes did not include information about nationality or country of origin. Such data was not gathered systematically by the researcher, giving us an overall, but not exact overview.

3   And increasingly so, based on national statistics for the health- and social sector in general, stating an increase in the work force of 7.4 percent of employed staff with a «foreign background» between 2013 and 2014 (www.ssb.no).

4   A substantial number of caring staff members have obtained the title of «registered nurse» from their country of origin. In most cases, these accreditations are not transferable to Norway and/or imply further training in Norway, which a minority «can afford», as they formulate it. A majority of caring staff members with foreign accreditation as «registered nurses» are given the title of «assisting nurse». Some, a minority, have or are undergoing further training to get accreditation in Norway.

5   Totaling 10 300 in 2014 for the entire health- and social sector in Norway, many of whom (close to 21 percent) are from Sweden (www.ssb.no). Interestingly there few Swedish (or from other parts of Western Europe, for that matter), assisting- or registered nurses employed at our nursing homes.

who do not speak properly. This leads to difficulties for the residents, families and collea-gues. Some residents, of course, become skeptical towards the lack of proper language and different colors, but we cannot choose them away because we are too few. (Unit leader, name of institution withheld).

While such sentiments were prevalent among many caring staff members and top administrators at our nursing home, they were not observed among residents, save for very few exceptions; most residents seemed either indiffe-rent or appreciative towards diversity among caring staff members, focusing on the *familiarity* of the caring staff member, rather than her country of origin or color of skin.

As a collective group, caring staff are dominant in nursing homes, dwarfing all other professional groups combined in sheer numbers. On average, the institutions in our sample have 70 caring staff members, including all caring staff in permanent positions (although with differing size of position), and excluding staff under temporary contracts, short-term temporary staff and students on internships. The total number of caring staff varies from 27 to 159, depending primarily on the number of residents in the institutions and the average size of positions in the respective nursing homes.

More relevant than the total number of caring staff is the *composition* of the respective professional groups and the number of caring staff relative to the number of residents. Not taking into account size of positions (percentage of full positions), registered nurses constitute 21 percent of total caring staff on average[6] (ranging from 14 to 40 percent). The percentage of registered nurses out of total staff is fairly similar from institution to institution, with one excep-tion: Galactic Manor, which actively prioritizes having registered nurses on duty on evening and night-shifts. The average percentage of assisting nurses (not taking into account the size of position) is 43 of total caring staff[7] (ranging from 32 to 63 percent, where the latter is disproportionally high). Assisting nurses are the largest professional group when combining figures for all six nursing homes. The percentage of assisting nurses measured against total number of caring staff varies more between institutions than for registered nurses. This can be connected to varying institutional practices when it comes

---

6   The national average for the entire health- and care sector in 2014 was 35 percent (www.helsenorge.no).

7   Similar to the national average of 40 percent in 2014 (www.helsenorge.no).

to offering assisting nurses part-time and/or temporary positions, as opposed to registered nurses who generally have large, in many cases full-time, permanent positions (see later). Assistants constitute 36 percent of total caring staff for all six nursing homes[8] (ranging from 11 to 46 percent). Again, there are large variations between institutions, which can be connected to size of positions, but also to differing practices related to a financial incentive of employing assistants rather than groups with more formal education. Such an incentive is manifested in differing practices of employing assistants in temporary positions, ranging from none, to some, to all assistants in temporary positions.

In nursing homes within the sample, in the municipality in general and in Norway, women are the majority; both residents and staff are predominantly female. Residents within our sample are between 70 and 90 percent female, while caring staff are almost exclusively female. On average, our nursing homes employ two male caring staff members in different types of positions. Although nursing homes are «gendered» institutions and work environments, for reasons of limitation the theme will not be discussed. Gender is still encompassed in the analysis, implicitly, for instance regarding «the hardship and toil» at the nursing home (Chapter 8), and has been covered extensively.

Another topic that speaks about nursing homes as a typical female-dominated work environment is the overall size of position for all caring staff at all institutions: 55 percent. Many caring staff members, especially assisting nurses and assistants, would prefer, if possible, larger positions, while pointing out that management will not offer full-time positions to better suit their needs relating to the overall shift-plans for the institutions. Although the nursing homes vary somewhat (as we shall see) concerning the respective size of positions, full-time positions for assisting nurses and assistants are considered rare and attractive. Management and a minority of caring staff members would typically argue that the low average size of position is a result of employers being flexible and offering positions suited to individual needs. A substantial number of assistants and some assisting nurses, meanwhile, are employed in temporary positions (often for a small number of hours). As mentioned, our nursing homes vary regarding the use of temporary positions, as they did in providing data of such use. Regretfully, the data on this is severely lacking, and should be added to by accounts from several administrators, pointing out that

---

8   Higher than the national average of 25 percent in 2014 (www.helsenorge.no).

assistants and, to some degree, assisting nurses are employed on temporary contracts out of necessity, in part caused by sick- and maternity leave. Contrary to such sentiments, administrators at Cloud House and Emerald Gardens stated that all positions were permanent, while data from Acre Woods and Durmstrang suggest relative low figures for *total* number of temporary positions: 11 and 6 percent respectively[9].

The average size of positions at our nursing homes ranges from 51 to 72 percent. Acre Woods, by far the largest institution, has the lowest average size of position, while Emerald Gardens has the highest average size by far. The latter can be explained by the respective nursing homes' practice of employing assistants in far higher positions than other nursing homes (average size of position for assistants for the other five nursing homes is relatively low – see later – thus decreasing the total average for size of position). The average size of position for the respective professional groups is 76 percent for registered nurses, 68 percent for assisting nurses and 26 percent for assistants[10]. The average size of position for registered nurses is generally high for all nursing homes, but also varies among them, ranging from 57 to 87 percent. Average size of position for assisting nurses is more evenly distributed between institutions, ranging from 60 to 79 percent. The nursing home with the lowest average size of position, Galactic Manor, has relatively few assisting nurses in their employ as a result of having disproportionally many registered nurses employed (see above). The average size of position for assistants is similar across institutions, ranging from 19 to 31 percent for five of the nursing homes, while the remaining, Emerald Gardens, averages 64 percent. It should be noted that size of position for assistants, although similar in total figures for most institutions, varies significantly internally; usually a few experienced assistants have large or full positions, while many, (university students working weekends, for instance) have very small positions. For many assistants, as opposed to most registered nurses or assisting nurses, small positions are considered ideal.

Both total and institutional numbers for the respective professional groups, as well as size of positions, are interesting in themselves, but have limited

---

9   For the remaining two nursing homes, data was not provided. At Galactic Manor, temporary positions were used extensively especially for assistants and assisting nurses who, in many cases would hold two or more temporary positions at the same time, making data difficult to generate.

10   Although technically not a «professional» group, assistants will, for simplicities sake, be described as such.

relevance when not taking the number of residents into account. All positions within what has been categorized as caring staff, amount to 232.1 full-time positions when combined. Total caring staff full-time positions amount to 0.879 positions per resident in total. In other words; there is almost one full-time position, either registered nurse, assisting nurse or assistant, for each nursing home resident. It should be kept in mind though that the 232.1 full-time positions are spread relatively «thinly» over 422 actual positions, most of which are part-time. In other words, *the nursing home resident sees many faces and feels many hands on a daily basis.*

The institutional average of full-time caring staff positions per resident varies somewhat between the six institutions, ranging from 0.72 to 1.07 full-time equivalents. The anomalies are to be found at each end of the spectrum, while the other four nursing homes have a similar coverage of caring staff per resident. An interesting point should be made about the two anomalies, Galactic Manor (highest) and Emerald Gardens (lowest). Although opposites for our sample when considering coverage of caring staff per resident, these are the two institutions that most closely resemble each other when considering general characteristics. Galactic Manor and Emerald Gardens are the only two small private non-profit nursing homes in our sample, and have almost the same number of residents. It should also be noted that the nursing home with the highest level of total staffing (Galactic Manor) also has the highest number of registered nurses.

The average number of full-time positions of registered nurses per resident for all six institutions is 0.26. For each full-time registered nurse, there are four residents on average, in other words. The coverage of registered nurses per resident varies significantly between institutions, ranging from 0.14 to 0.54 full-time registered nurses per resident. Even when excluding the largest anomaly (Galactic Manor), the nursing home with the highest coverage of registered nurses per resident has a coverage of more than twice that of the lowest. The total number of full-time assisting nurses per resident for all six institutions amounts to 0.51. There is moderate variation between the institutions (ranging from 0.37 to 0.57). Total and respective numbers for assisting nurses should be read in conjunction with the coverage for registered nurses: nursing homes with better coverage of registered nurses tend to have lesser coverage of assisting nurses and vice versa. Assistants, as opposed to registered nurses and assisting nurses, are a small group both in total numbers and in number of full-time positions per resident. In total, there are 0.15 assistants employed per resident, while there is a significant institutional difference, ranging from 0.07 to 0.28.

Age of caring staff is perhaps mostly relevant when seen in relation to experience, especially in our context. Age should still be mentioned, since there are distinct patterns within each professional group. The average age for all caring staff is 41 years old. The average age of registered nurses is 42 years, of assisting nurses 46 years and 41 years for assistants. There is remarkably small variation between institutions; all follow the pattern of assistants, registered nurses and assisting nurses in ascending order of age, while the relative difference between the groups is similar for all nursing homes. It should be noted that while registered nurses and assisting nurses are relatively homogeneous in age, assistants vary significantly, from 18 to 67 years old.

Experience, measured in tenure at the respective institutions[11], varies greatly between professional groups and between institutions. Caring staff have an average level of experience of 7 years and 10 months, when including all institutions[12]. In other words; experience can be considered generally high, especially when considering that only tenure from the current institution is included. Total, average experience for all staff varied between institutions from 4 years and 1 month and 12 years and 7 months. Galactic Manor is the nursing home with the lowest average level of experience, in all likelihood explained by being a relatively newly built institution. It is interesting to note that the two nursing homes with the largest variation in total staffing and in total caring staff per resident, Galactic Manor (high) and Emerald Gardens (low), are the two nursing homes with the highest average level of experience; 10 years and 6 months for Galactic Manor and 12 years of 7 months for Emerald Gardens. In the case of Emerald Gardens, it seems that total level of staffing is not a significant factor for rate of turnover, perhaps contrary to popular belief.

---

11   *As continuity* at the respective institutions will be a significant focus in the analysis, I chose to limit tenure to present institution, rather than nursing homes or the health sector in general.

12   Regretfully, I was only able to gather a tenure list for staff at four of the six institutions. While all institutions were willing to offer anonymized information about tenure, only four had such information stored electronically, and were able to provide it. One institution did have the data on written, individualized personnel files (which I opted out of viewing), while another simply did not have the information.

Experience within the respective professional groups follows a distinct pattern: assisting nurses have the longest experience by far (11 years and 9 months when combining all nursing homes), followed by registered nurses (6 years and 7 months) and assistants (3 years and 3 months). All included nursing homes follow this pattern. Assisting nurses are highly experienced at all nursing homes included, a point I will return to in the analysis, exemplified with the average level of experience of 15 years and 5 months at Emerald Gardens. Registered nurses are generally also highly experienced, but differ considerably within each institution; some are new, some have been at the nursing homes for many years.

To summarize, caring staff at our nursing homes have a relatively high level of experience and knowledge from within their respective units and nursing homes, but not a high degree of stability, in the form of full-time positions. This will be a central element in the analysis: many caring staff members do not work in the respective nursing homes as regularly as possible (for them) or perhaps as would be ideal (for the residents). Many caring staff members say that such a situation is not ideal: assisting nurses with smaller percentages of full-time positions state that they would prefer larger positions. As a general rule, registered nurses are more often offered full-time positions and/or can have a size of position in accordance with their individual preference, while many assistants would prefer only to work part-time. Our nursing homes, then, employ many caring staff members, perhaps more than ideal, as opposed to prioritizing *stability* of staff.

Measuring levels of physician coverage at the respective nursing homes proved a difficult task, as all nursing homes have different arrangements with their physicians including (for most) a great deal of flexibility with regards to time spent at the nursing homes and availability outside time spent at the nursing homes. Reliable data on physician coverage was provided from three of the nursing homes. For the remaining three, data on physician coverage was gathered, but as its accuracy is uncertain, this data will not be included. At Acre Woods, two physicians are employed by the institution, totaling 0.39 physician hours per week, per resident (that is approximately 20 minutes per resident per week). At Durmstrang, employing a consultant, physician hours per week amount to 0.27 (approximately 15 minutes). Both of these figures are calculated based on *actual* time spent at the nursing homes. Additionally, physicians at both nursing homes were available by phone outside these hours (for

Durmstrang, at all hours, also including sporadic visitations outside the allotted time). At Emerald Gardens, which employed a physician through the municipality (even though Emerald Gardens is a private institution), time spent at the nursing home for the physician amounted to 0.19 (approximately 12 minutes) hours per week, per resident. The physician was available most hours outside of visiting day, an arrangement not always taken advantage of, according to caring staff. At the other nursing homes, physicians will spend parts of a given day at the nursing homes, between approximately two and six hours, depending on the day. The three nursing homes varied considerably regarding contact with physicians outside time spent at the nursing homes, some stating that the physician was not always available, implying that they had to contact emergency wards instead. In general, time actually spent at the nursing homes *and* availability outside time spent at the nursing homes vary considerably, and should be viewed as mutually relevant.

The *types of employment* for physicians, in contrast to hours worked, is more easily available and can be said to vary considerably within our sample of nursing homes. The variation is connected to ownership and size of nursing homes. As mentioned, public (and some private) nursing homes employ physicians through the municipality, who perform obligatory duty work in nursing homes. The two public institutions, Cloud House and Coruscant, and two of the private institutions, Galactic Manor and Emerald Gardens, did so. Acre Woods employed physicians directly, while Durmstrang employed a physician as a private consultant (the physician in question worked exclusively as a consultant for nursing homes, as opposed to alternating between work in nursing homes and as a general practitioner). Although our sample is far too small to generalize on the matter, type of employment seems to be connected to size of institution (as well as ownership); larger (private) institutions tend to employ physicians directly. Being a small institution, Durmstrang is an exception to this tendency. Type of employment of physician seems also, again based on our limited sample, to be related to number of hours contracted to the position. At the nursing homes employing physicians directly, Acre Woods and Durmstrang, physicians have more contracted hours (relative to number of residents), *and* spend more of their time in the nursing home. *Overall* time spent at a nursing home for physicians (as opposed to hours per resident), should also be seen as significant, for instance with regards to collaboration with caring staff, as will be argued (Chapter 10). Both overall and relative (to number of residents) time spent in nursing homes can, however, be problematic to ascertain, as physicians' *intended* and *actual* time in nursing homes might differ, and because physicians have different arrangements with nursing homes as to if and how they can be contacted outside office hours.

Staffing levels for caring staff, and coverage and types of employment for physicians will be treated, in the following discussions, as significant for practices of hospitalization. *The ways* in which they are significant, meanwhile, might be indirect and involved, and might also vary between institutions.

3.3.3. Actual coverage of staff

While a description of the number of caring staff per resident can provide an indication of *intended coverage* at the respective institution, it is not necessarily equal to *actual coverage* of caring staff, as demonstrated in detail elsewhere (Jacobsen 2005: 43). Actual coverage of caring staff is difficult to measure, as all nursing homes have several and different ways of filling vacancies, and no procedures to measure actual coverage.

All six nursing homes have intricate shift plans, describing not only the division of the respective shifts, but also many variations within a shift, the preparation of which takes a large part of the unit leadership's time. The shift plans are intricate and complicated for several reasons. The total number of staff employed is high, even for the smallest nursing homes; the shift plan has to adhere to relatively strict national work regulations (in contrast to the form of other regulations); many caring staff members have less than full-time positions; and there is a relatively high level of short-and long term sickness absence in addition to maternity- and other forms of leave. Data on sick leave was only provided by one nursing home, Acre Woods, registering 10.4 days per full-time position annually, on average, while I did not obtain data on the level of different types of leave.

The occurrence of sickness absence and regular staff on leave makes shift plans not only difficult to construct, but also difficult to maintain; short-term sickness absence, especially, cannot be planned for, making filling vacant positions a constant battle at all nursing homes.

Evening-shift at Emerald Gardens: At the start of the evening-shift most of the shift workers were present at 14.00, even though they were supposed to start later. Two of the day-shift workers, including the unit leader, remained even though their shift had ended. The other day-shift workers had already left. As the first part of the evening-shift was relatively quiet, most of the staff gathered at the nurses' station, preparing themselves for the shift or talking privately amongst themselves. The two who had remained from the day-shift worked diligently on getting staff to cover for vacancies the next day. One of them, the unit leader, was on the phone, while the other, an assisting nurse, went through a telephone list of possible temporary staff (to my understanding, a list of known temporary staff who had worked at the nursing home on some occasion). When they did not succeed, they discussed who of the regular staff could potentially cover the vacant shifts the following day. After about twenty minutes, they still had not found anyone to fill the positions. The two decided to call it a day and leave, after discussing the matter with one of the assisting nurses on evening-shift, who took over the job. Meanwhile, three other caring staff members had gathered at a table in the nurses' station, going through their respective shift plans, figuring out when they were on shift the coming week and discussing when the different day-shifts (six in total) started and ended. The assisting nurse given the job of filling the next day's vacancies said she had to try calling later, because it was too time consuming to do now. Before leaving for other tasks, she explained that the shift plans were complicated and difficult to fill, especially during the summer. *It is difficult to get temps when they too are on summer holiday. I´ve had to work all summer, and have taken so many extra shifts, even though I only have a 69 percent position. It is difficult to say no.*

The six nursing homes all have different routines when it comes to filling temporary vacancies. Some use temporary staff agencies either exclusively or in part (considered expensive, but reliable), some have lists of former students and others who have volunteered to be used as temporary staff, while all nursing homes must relate to the dilemma of whether or not to fill temporary vacancies at all. All six nursing homes combine the use of either temporary agencies or known replacements with the practice of not filling temporary vacancies[13]. As explained by a unit leader (Acre Woods):

Here at the home everyone is known. We usually have temps every day; there is no way around that. A large bulk are regular «call temps». They only work here, so all in all mainly the same ones. We also use those who only have weekend positions; they tend to

---

13 The tendency of not filling vacancies, arbitrarily or systematically, was not found in a study on patterns of sickness absence representative for all nursing homes in Norway (Holmeide & Eimot 2010: 8). I believe that this might be attributed to the fact that respondents do not report not filling vacancies when asked, thus participant observation at nursing homes is better suited than a survey to uncover such discrepancies.

be students. The thing is that it doesn't pay to call in new people, it takes too long. It is not worth it, and you can just as well not call at all. But sometimes we have to call, because no one can get paid overtime[14], no one shall exceed more than 35 hours on average, and the same goes for shifts that are altered. The exception is when registered nurses get sick in the evenings. Then they have to cover. Sometimes we have to step in and take over.

A common trait for all nursing homes when replacing caring staff members, either for short- or long-term sickness absence, holidays or shorter leaves, is the tendency of replacing a caring staff member with members from a lower (in terms of formal education) professional category: a registered nurse is replaced by an assisting nurse, and an assisting nurse is replaced by an assistant. This practice seems to be a common trait for nursing homes in Norway and elsewhere (see also Holmeide & Eimot 2010). The practice can be explained by the fact that caring staff with formal education, especially registered nurses, are difficult to get as temporary staff:

Registered nurses work full time positions, usually at hospitals. If they want to work in nursing homes at all, they don't want small percentages, or just temporary work; they want full-time, permanent positions (Unit leader, Cloud House).

The challenge of maintaining the intended shift plan, which in itself can be said to include only a minimum of needed coverage (see Chapter 8), is shared among all six nursing homes. They differ, however, in how they cope with this challenge; some use known replacements, others use outsiders. The nursing homes also differ when it comes to if and how often they chose not to fill temporary vacancies, as mentioned. This is a difference of degree, however; all six nursing homes have chosen not to fill temporary vacancies at some point, but differ greatly when it comes to how often. Still, the problem is universal for the nursing homes; they all experience short- and long-term absences that are difficult to plan for and are difficult to get adequate coverage for, resulting in more strain on the staff not absent and, more importantly, the residents.

Monday morning, undisclosed nursing home. There are only three caring staff members present, two have called in sick, and they have not been able to get anyone to cover yet, an assisting nurse explains in a relatively calm moment after breakfast: *But*

---

14   Referring to regular staff and the possibility for them to cover temporary vacancies.

we shall see, there is still time. The assisting nurse, having a cup of coffee while looking strained, tells me that she has been working all weekend: *It was tiresome. Just one of those times, I guess.* She paused before continuing: *We were supposed to be four, but one of them called in sick at 6.30!*[15] *So we had to be three during the entire weekend. They tried calling, but it didn't work.* Another pause, while drinking coffee and exchanging words with a resident sitting next to her: *It was so busy the whole time. We didn't even have time to eat. I work every other weekend, and this is the third time in a row this has happened.*

As described, the types of employment and size of positions vary considerably for physicians, more so than the general composition of caring staff. At some larger nursing homes physicians are employed at close to or full-time positions by the institutions, while physicians at smaller nursing homes, strictly speaking, are working compulsory time away from their primary employment. Related to their mode of employment, it will be argued that the communication and collaboration between caring staff and physicians also vary considerably. Similarly, and relationally, the amount and forms of communication *outside office hours* between caring staff and physicians vary considerably.

At Acre Woods and Durmstrang, caring staff could contact physicians at their own convenience; in the evening and at weekends for instance. At Durmstrang, the physician was also available at night and on holidays. The remaining four nursing homes had other, more limited arrangements with their physicians; either in the form of no contact outside office hours (physicians could be contacted at their physician's office during office hours, if available, but not at other times), or at certain specific times. At most of these nursing homes the physician could be contacted outside hours spent at the nursing homes, but were often difficult to reach. At one nursing home, for instance, the physician would return calls after 15.00, in many cases several hours after a potentially acute incident. Consequently, caring staff in the respective nursing homes adopted different procedures as to whether or not they contacted the physicians´ services at the emergency ward or not, and to what degree they were directly involved in communication and collaboration with family.

---

15   Indicating, in my opinion, that this was very late.

The difference between *intended* and *actual* coverage of physicians also seems to vary within our sample, although more on an individual rather than systemic level. For several of our nursing homes, the institutions are allocated one day of physicians' services per week, while physicians would spend somewhere between a couple of hours and a full day effectively in the nursing homes, depending on a multitude of factors, including travel time, number of residents considered acute or demanding, and the swiftness of the visitation rounds. Particularly at two smaller nursing homes, weekly variations in time spent by physicians was pointed out by nursing home staff. Such a practice is contrary to that of Acre Woods, where the two physicians are employed locally, and spend their allocated time in the nursing home, as is also the case for the smaller nursing home employing a consultant for relatively few residents. In general, then, physicians employed in smaller positions through the municipality did not always spend their allocated time in the institutions, while physicians being contracted more hours per resident by the nursing homes (or as a consultant) did. Consequently, *measuring* actual coverage of physicians, proved a difficult task; in part because of the periodic variations at the respective nursing homes, in part because of the different arrangements of (and different execution of) contact outside time spent at the nursing homes. Some of the nursing homes, for example, call the emergency ward for all incidents happening after 16.00; some call occasionally and at different times; some only call on very rare occasions (during their physician's holiday, for instance). Calling the emergency ward, regardless of how often, is to a varying degree considered a lesser alternative than the attending physician is. In nursing homes employing a physician directly, caring staff consider the level of knowledge at the emergency ward, both of the specific resident and of the patient group in general, to be far less than that of their physician. For caring staff in nursing homes employing physicians in smaller positions, this sentiment varies; at two nursing homes in particular, no difference in competence and knowledge between nursing home and emergency ward physicians was expressed.

3.3.4. The residents

The multi-faceted and dynamic relationships between residents and staff will be presented and discussed throughout this analysis. As background information, it might therefore be beneficial to have an overview of the general characteristics of residents from the sample[16]. The overview should, however, be read carefully, as it provides a general description of combined characteristics, without emphasizing relative variations within the respective categories used.

The average age of all residents in Acre Woods is 89.2 years. Residents in dementia units are on average younger (86.6 years in average) than others. 71 percent of all residents are considered to have dementia[17]. Interestingly, only 93 percent of residents in dementia units are considered to have dementia. 79 percent of residents suffer from incontinence[18]. 84 percent of residents are considered to «eat independently»[19], while 50 percent are considered to «walk independently»[20]. For the latter two categories, residents from dementia units scored significantly higher compared to other residents. Only six percent of all residents are considered to be able to wash themselves, while eight percent are considered to be able to dress themselves. Six percent of residents were considered to be «partly or completely bedridden» (none from the dementia unit).

Overall, but excluding the dementia unit, resident groups are strikingly similar from one unit to the next. For all categories, with minor exceptions for incontinence and the ability to wash independently (slightly higher in one unit for both categories), units appear to have a similar composition of residents. Average age, for instance, only varies by 0.3 years, between the somatic units.

Although reasonably indicative of the general characteristics of nursing home residents, data such as these fail to demonstrate the variation of nursing home residents, especially when it comes to alertness, speech and ability to communicate with staff. An example, taken from my very first visit to a new unit, can illustrate such a variation, although it should be mentioned that the

---

16   Data for resident characteristics were difficult to get access to and time-consuming to analyze. None of the nursing homes had generated overall data for all residents, but rather individualized data stored on electronic or written personal journals. Getting access to these would imply breaching the ethical approval for the project. I therefore opted to gather generalized data on residents for one of the nursing homes, Acre Woods. The data was obtained by interviewing unit leaders, who either knew the information sought after, or provided it through the journals, in an anonymized form. As such, no data that could be connected to specific residents was given.

17   Based on the discretion of unit leaders, rather than electronic journals. Journals are not always updated, as evident both at our nursing homes and elsewhere. Selbæk (et al. 2007: 846) found that only 55 percent of residents suffering from dementia had the diagnosis registered in their electronic journals.

18   Some of which might be continent during day-time, but not at night (when they wear diapers).

19   Defined as «the ability to eat a majority of the meal independently, rather than being fed, if the meal is prepared and presented in an adequate manner».

20   Including the ability to walk independently with aids (such as «walking frames»).

protagonist, Anny, is not your average nursing home resident (if such a thing exists):

> Morning at Coruscant. One registered nurse, two assisting nurses and one nursing student are in the unit attending to the residents before, during and after breakfast. The residents are at different stages of their morning routines; some are eating, some are being prepared for breakfast in their rooms; while some are waiting for staff to attend them. I am «guided» by an assisting nurse to one of the residents sitting alone while eating breakfast (*Sit with her. She is good to talk to*, which I interpret to mean that she is among the more vocal and «present» residents). Anny, the resident, is indeed very present, clear, positive and sharing, and when introduced to me *as a visitor learning about the nursing home* she continuously boasts about the nursing home: *It is wonderful here! Everything is nice. Can you imagine being served food all the time and even getting help with getting ready and everything, it's like a hotel*, she says while smiling enthusiastically. She fixes the scarf covering her hair and apologizes for not being properly groomed: *You see, I have an appointment with the hairdresser later.* Meanwhile, another resident, Maria, sitting in a wheelchair close to Anny, has been uneasy and upset, trying to get contact with either residents or staff. Maria has been shouting *hello* constantly, at least every 20 seconds. The staff have alternated between disregarding her, and giving her short replies asking her to calm down, apparently used to her calls. Maria seems, in my eyes, fragile and very dependent on help, apparently not able to move her arms, feet or even her head, or able to articulate anything besides *hello*. Finally, Anny, has had enough: *You need to stop bugging us now*, she says in a stern, almost maternal tone, obviously accustomed to being in charge. A short while later, an assisting nurse accompanies Maria back to her room where she remains alone. Anny moves to a sofa in the corner after fetching a novel in her room, and proceeds to read for about half an hour.

3.3.5. Families[21] and volunteers

As a general point, families of residents will be mentioned throughout, when deemed relevant to understanding the practices of the caring staff. Families of residents *are* important for the practices of caring staff, particularly when residents

---

21   «Family» will be used as a collective term covering «next of kin», «relatives» and «visitors» (visits by others than family members were rare at our nursing homes, but are still included for the sake of simplicity), also combining the Norwegian terms «familie», «pårørende» and «besøkende».

become acutely or severely ill (Bottrell et al. 2001, see also Chapter 4). Caring staff relate to families, explicitly and implicitly, and formally and informally. As will be discussed later, nursing homes relate *differently* to families, especially concerning if, how and when issues concerning potential illnesses are discussed. Some of the nursing homes have formalized routines regarding when and how such issues are addressed. Not all do, however, while some do not always follow their formalized routines. Our nursing homes also vary considerably regarding documentation of families' preferences for treatment and potential hospitalizations; from systematized to almost random. The difficulties discussing end of life with family members of loved ones as well as the difference in approach towards families can be illustrated by how staff talk about their meetings with them:

I think that it is difficult to address, that is; discussing the end when they have just arrived, but still it is important. We are good at it and prioritize it too. Sometimes it can depend on the individual, the family I mean; some are easier than others, and some have a clearer idea of what they want. But usually it is fine. At the end, it works nicely. Especially the physician, who is part of the conversations, can get the families to understand what we think. (Nursing home administrator, Durmstrang).

Some are more ambivalent towards family members, conveying a mismatch of expectations between the family and the institution:

Well, it sort of works. But it is a work in progress, sometimes our wishes don't correspond. And I think that's because of all the negative stuff about nursing homes in the media, newspapers and news; they influence how relatives view who we are as health workers. Then they see us in a certain way, and I feel that they might not trust our competence. They can be on guard towards us. And I think this has changed, just within the last five years, how they see us. How shall I say this so it doesn't come out all negative, because it really is positive that they are involved, I'm not sure, but it can be challenging. But on the other hand, if they really are involved, then they demand more from us, and we have to be ready, and we cannot simply say «Oh well, they are really tiresome, those relatives.» (Unit leader, Cloud House).

Notwithstanding the general importance of family members for the potential treatment of residents and the differences in approach towards families, families at our nursing homes are still not a prominent part of everyday life (see also Hauge 2004). While a few residents received visitors almost every day, most rarely received visitors and many never received any. At any given time when entering any of our nursing homes, the likelihood of a visitor being present was far lower than them not being present. The nursing homes are places for residents and staff, conceptually (see Chapter 7.1) and in reality. Visitors, in general, do not impact on the mundanity and regularity of nursing home life. An exception to this tendency might illustrate the point, by the reactions of staff and residents to such a rare occasion:

> Coruscant, May 16th (the day before the national holiday of Norway): The administration at the nursing home have made arrangements with the neighboring kindergarten so that the children will walk past the nursing home in a traditional parade. As the kindergarten is closed on the 17th, they are visiting one day early. At one of the units, residents and staff alike are ready and excited. At about 10.30 all residents in the unit are gathered in the common room carrying flags and looking out the window. Even a bedridden resident has been wheeled in. Most smile, anticipating the arrival of the children, while a few doze off. Four caring staff members are present, visibly excited. When they see the children arriving, the unit leader makes an impulsive decision, opens the door to the garden area outside and shouts towards the adults accompanying the children, asking them to please walk through the unit and not just pass it by. They comply. About 40 children walk through the unit, cheering and waving their flags. The spectacle is over in just three minutes. One of the caring staff members, an assisting nurse, is crying, while two others have tears in their eyes. Most of the residents are smiling and several are talking about «the beautiful children». The rare occasion became the talk of the unit for weeks to come.

In the same way as family, volunteers also do not influence the everyday life at our nursing homes to a high degree. Nursing homes in Norway have, in general, fewer volunteers than their international counterparts, related to the position of the public sector within Norwegian healthcare. Only one of our nursing homes – Emerald Gardens - had volunteers contributing on a regular basis, while most others had volunteers, mostly in the form of entertainment, contributing sporadically.

Although family members of residents do not generally influence the everyday life in our nursing homes, I will argue that they – by the ways they are approached and engaged – are highly influential for practices of hospitalization. As we will return to: family might not explain overall rates of hospitalization, but can contribute to an understanding of how and why nursing homes differ in practices of hospitalization.

3.4. A brief introduction to the empirical phenomenon of hospitalizations

For a six month period all hospitalizations of residents (or rather «transfers from the nursing home to hospitals») were registered by caring staff at Acre Woods. The data was meant to be a supplement to the qualitative data on decisions of hospitalization, by providing an overview of the overall occurrence of hospitalizations at the nursing home, and by providing added information from units in which the researcher did not spend much time. As such, the data did not cover *potential* but rather *actual* hospitalizations. Despite this problematic aspect, and methodological faults, to which we will return, the data provided some insight into further areas of study. In other words, the data did not provide clear answers, but did raise new questions.

The information was registered on forms detailing time of transfer, type of transportation, reason for transfer, and, if available, effect of transfer (what happened to the resident). Each unit, through the unit leader or assisting leader, was responsible for filling out the forms, which facilitated an analysis of potential differences between units. All transfers from nursing homes to hospitals, including non-acute, were included, with the aim of providing an overview of the different variants potentially defined as hospitalizations.

While all transportations from the nursing home to hospitals were supposed to be registered within the six month period, they were, in all likelihood, not. Although the respective units were reminded of the forms every week, a majority of them seemed not to prioritize them, although they would not express such a lack of interest to the researcher. Generally, as will be discussed in Chapter 8, caring staff in nursing homes are burdened with internal and external forms and registrations, from researchers and others, contributing to an amount of «paperwork» that adds to the already pressing total workload. Such tasks are not in compliance with the tasks considered ideal for caring staff (at least as conveyed by themselves). As such, new forms to be filled in are not welcomed, contributing to, in all probability, a lack of reporting for most of the units. One unit, meanwhile, took a different approach than the others; *our unit* was far more diligent in their reporting than others, probably because the researcher was there most days, reminding them, explicitly and through simply being there, of the registrations. Consequently, *our unit* reported far more transfers than any other unit, even more than all the other units combined (a paradox, considering the emphasis from caring staff at *our unit* on not to hospitalize its residents, see Chapter 10). As such, the registrations do not, in all probability, correspond with actual transfers, and should therefore be disregarded in terms of representativeness. Despite this, some general tendencies should be pointed out, as they point to potential tendencies that are interesting in themselves and relevant for future discussions.

Transfers to hospitals did not increase during the summer holidays, according to the data set. Considering the relative downsizing of overall staff, use of temporary staff and consequent lack of experienced staff (to be discussed in Chapter 10), this tendency was a surprising finding. Not surprising is the tendency of a disproportionate amount of transfers during the afternoon and evening, perhaps connected to the hectic nature of these shifts and the relative scarce staffing level. The amount of transfers during the afternoon and evening were also of a more acute nature, as appointments and check-ups at the hospitals took place earlier in the day. In contrast, there were few transfers during night-shifts, which were even more scarcely staffed than during afternoon and evening. Relatively few transportations during the morning hours would suggest that potential transfers during night-time were not postponed until the morning shift arrived, perhaps indicating that there were, in fact, few acute incidents during the night. Friday and Saturday saw an increase of hospitalizations, giving credence to the assumption of less staff leading to more acute transfers, while Sunday, surprisingly, saw less. However, more transfers were made (by appointment and not) on Monday than any other day, in accordance with the assumption of caring staff «waiting out» potential hospitalizations during scarcely staffed periods.

Although faulty through being based on self-reporting, the data-set still point to potential areas of further study, particularly pertaining to the significance of level of experience of staff.

Part one of the analysis: a preliminary analysis of hospitalizations from nursing homes

In these chapters, I will present and analyze how hospitalizations, as a theoretical construct *and* empirical phenomenon can be understood, and how the empirical phenomenon of hospitalization can, potentially, relate to various, interrelated factors.

First, research on hospitalizations from nursing homes will be presented and analyzed, from which areas or approaches that are not extensively covered will be isolated. I will argue that this study can be seen as a supplement to the presented research literature (representing a dominant doxa), by covering areas and approaches not extensively covered and adopted.

These areas, most notably a focus on potential rather than actual hospitalizations, the potential interrelatedness of conditions and factors influencing decisions, and the everyday practices of institutions will be addressed in Chapter 5 (analyzing how factors influence practices of hospitalization) and Chapter 6 (discussing understandings of the concept and the empirical phenomenon of «hospitalization»), laying the foundation for the discussions in Part Three of the analysis.

An analysis of the literature on hospitalization

Current and influential literature on the subject of hospitalizations from nursing homes will be presented to identify potential areas not extensively covered by the literature. By doing so, a presentation of the literature's findings (what it presents as influential for practices of hospitalization) will be given, but also an understanding of how and why studies are undertaken in a certain manner. Is there, in other words, a dominating doxa on this particular field of research?

As «*(…) every established order tends to produce (to very different degrees and with very different means) the naturalization of its own arbitrariness (…) the natural and social world appears as self-evident*» (Bourdieu 2012: 164), a dynamic synthesized by Bourdieu with the term «doxa». By our understanding, doxa is the silent consensus within a given field, pertaining to understandings, attitudes and knowledge commonly adopted and shared by agents as implicit mechanisms of making order of reality. Doxa is the underlying social coherence of a certain systemic composition, which transcends subjective intentions and conscious deliberations (Petersen & Callewaert 2013: 124), while taking the form of self-evidence and being undisputed (Bourdieu 2012: 164). It is largely taken for granted, not immediately visible, understandable or communicable by those possessing it.

Furthermore, doxa will, by my understanding, refer both to *content of meaning* and *mode of presentations*; that is, both to *what* is, more or less, taken for granted and to *how* it is presented. This latter aspect of doxa is not to be confused with the term «discourse», which is often applied. Bourdieu's term «*the universe of discourse*», refers to that which is or can (potentially) be discussed, including heterodoxa, imbedded *within* the field of doxa, or the universe of that which is undiscussed. Heterodoxa can be seen as a discourse but at the same time does not necessarily alter or influence doxa, as it remains bounded by the limitations set by it.

Doxic representations in the research literature will in this chapter be presented and analyzed in relation to orthodoxic (explicit maintenance of the dominating doxa) and heterodoxic (explicit deviations from doxa) representations, distinguishable from doxa by «(…) *implying awareness and recognition of the possibility of antagonistic beliefs*» (Bourdieu 2012: 164). As I will argue; there is a distinct, identifiable and dominating doxa within the research area (see also Ågotnes et al. 2015). Heterodoxic representations, meanwhile, can be found. Heterodoxic representations within the literature are, in part, incapable of «*problematizing all implicit preconditions*» (Petersen & Callewaert 2013: 124, my translation) of the dominant doxa, but also, in part, capable of bringing the undiscussed into discussion (Bourdieu 2012: 164).

The literature covering the topic of hospitalizations from nursing homes, explicitly or implicitly, is large in size and scope. For simplicity's sake I will therefore focus on literature addressing the specific topic of hospitalization from nursing homes as a main area of research, first internationally and then for Norway. As the research literature, even when only including literature explicitly focusing on hospitalizations, is extensive, most of the referenced studies will be presented briefly, by synthesizing content and approaches, without, I believe, simplifying.

4.1. International literature on hospitalization

«Hospitalization from nursing homes» has been a much studied topic for several decades, especially in North America. This emphasis can be attributed to a general consensus about the negative impact hospitalization has for those involved, both personally for the residents/patients and financially for the institutions (OIG 2013). Hospitalizations are, as we shall see, viewed as problematic, a view that is rarely contradicted, to the point of being cemented as a «*regime of truth*» (McCloskey & Hoonaard 2007). Consequently, a majority of the literature aims, explicitly or implicitly, to reduce the occurrence of hospitalization.

4.1.1. General characteristics

Overall, the research literature on hospitalization from nursing homes is strikingly similar in research design and methodology, although with some notable exceptions. A large majority of the research literature has the form of relatively short research articles published in medical and/or health oriented journals, and usually follow the structure and outline typical in the medical science field. Research articles typically use retrospective analysis of the occurrence of hospitalizations derived from large databases of patients, institutions and/or jurisdictions, resulting in a relatively large population sample. A majority of studies originate from North America, most from the U.S., where the topic of hospitalization has been a widely discussed topic for decades. Recently, other countries seem to be following suit. Typically, in the case of the U.S., the population sample incudes one or several federal states, as opposed to a city, county or smaller region. The population sample is typically analyzed in accordance with one or several corresponding factors, respectively. For instance, the population sample, «hospitalizations from nursing homes in Texas», can be measured against institutional numbers, for example of «size», «number of registered nurses hours per resident per day», «number of Medicaid patients», and/or «number of residents over 85 years of age». The factors are then analyzed in accordance with relevance for hospitalization, and typically ascribed a strength of correlation; «size» might be considered to be significantly correlated to level of hospitalization, while «coverage of registered nurses» is considered to be moderately significant. The potential significance of the connection between the respective independent variables is, as will be shown in more detail later, seldom studied. Some studies do, however, break with the commonly adopted designs and approaches, adding valuable and supplementary insight to the object of study.

Hospitalization can, as will be discussed, be defined as an event occurring when a resident of a nursing home is transferred to a hospital or an emergency ward, either planned or acute, for some form of medical treatment. While some of the research makes a point of separating transfers from nursing homes to a) hospitals and b) emergency wards, and some separate a) planned hospitalizations and b) acute hospitalizations, far from all do. An operationalization or a definition of «hospitalization» is often missing, while those who do operationalize or define do not always concur. Even though definitions of what constitutes a hospitalization differ or are absent (Castle & Mor 1996), research articles still refer to overall numbers for hospitalizations. Typically these are overall average rates within a given geographical area (Ibid., Grabowski et al. 2008, Brooks et al. 1994, Godden & Pollock 2001, Graverholt et al. 2011, Stephens et al. 2011). To simplify, two literature reviews can be used, supplemented by a governmental report to illustrate how rates of hospitalization are presented. In the first literature review, (Castle & Mor 1996) national (U.S) estimates ranged from 25 to 49 percent annual hospitalization rates. In the second review (Grabowski et al. 2008), estimates ranged between 9 and 59 percent annual hospitalization rates. In a national report (U.S.) from the Office of the Inspector General, annual hospitalization rates varied from less than 1 to 69.7 percent, with an average of 25 percent (OIG 2013).

Rates of hospitalization, then, appear to differ between institutions. To use the second review as an example: the probability of being hospitalized varies 6.5 times from lowest to highest. Some articles have also argued that variations in rates of hospitalizations differ between institutions within smaller geographical areas (Carter 2003a). The variations within smaller geographical areas are not taken into account for a large part of the research literature, particularly segments focusing on patient characteristics.

4.1.2. What is the problem?

Why is hospitalization, even given the premise that its occurrence is relatively high and that nursing homes' practices might vary, a relevant topic for research? Most research articles answer this question by stating that hospitalization for many patients is not beneficial (Ackermann 2001, Anphalahan & Gibson 2008, Boockvar et al. 2005, Creditor 1993, Fried & Mor 1997, Intrator et al. 1999, Intrator et al. 2004, Konetzka et al. 2008, Ouslander & Berenson 2011, Read 1999), and that a significant portion of them should not have taken place. To be specific: in many cases, hospitalization leads to a worsening of functional abilities, even though the specific ailment for which one is hospitalized improves (Creditor 1993):

> «Hospitalization and bed rest superimpose factors such as enforced immobilization, reduction of plasma volume, accelerated bone loss, increased closing volume, and sensory deprivation. Any of these factors may thrust vulnerable older persons into a state of irreversible functional decline.» (Grabowski et al. 2008)

Few articles deal directly with *why* unwarranted hospitalizations occur (Fried & Mor 1997), but rather focus on the potential occurrence of them. Research articles are typically concerned with whether or not hospitalizations may be unnecessary or unwanted, either in general (Grabowski et al. 2008,

O'Malley et al. 2007, Walker et al. 2009), for specific conditions such as infections (Boockvar et al. 2005), pneumonia (Dosa 2005) or dementia (Stephens et al. 2011, Phelan et al. 2012), or for unwanted (side) effects of hospitalization, often defined as «iatrogenic complications» (Fried & Mor 1997). It is thought that if the patient can receive the same treatment and care at the nursing home, the iatrogenic complications, such as *relocation stress syndrome»* (Castle 2001b, Intrator et al. 1999), pressure ulcers and delirium, (Dosa 2005, Konetzka et al. 2008) can be avoided.

The definition of what constitutes an «avoidable» or «potentially preventable» hospitalization and which conditions are included in such a definition differ between researchers (Grabowski et al. 2008, Vossius et al. 2013). Also the *occurrence* of such hospitalizations varies in the literature. Despite such a variation, ranging from 7.8 percent (Vossius et al. 2013) to 67 percent (Ouslander et al. 2010), the research literature seems to concur that the occurrence of avoidable hospitalizations is unwarrantedly high, with very few exceptions (Jensen et al. 2009). There is also relative agreement on which conditions are the most likely to lead to an avoidable hospitalization. Most frequently mentioned are congestive heart failure (40 percent) and pneumonia (35 percent) (Pappas & Hadden 1997). Jablonski et al. (2007) criticize the research majority's understanding of avoidable hospitalization, stating that many overemphasize occurrences because of «(…) *the use of specific research designs and methods that do not include the whole «story» of the transfer decisions»* (267). In short it is argued that because of the selected research designs, most commonly the use of *«chart reviews»* (Ibid.), or *«retrospective record reviews»* (McCloskey & Hoonaard 2007), the analysis of the actual decision making process is not taken into account.

To summarize, nursing homes hospitalize a lot, and they hospitalize differently. Hospitalization is understood as unnecessary or unwarranted for many patients. We have, in other words, a different way of operating for something that is not beneficial or at least ambiguous in effect. It seems, in a majority of the research literature, to follow that someone, somewhere is over-treated. If not, someone somewhere is undertreated, but given the high annual hospitalization rates, this seems more unlikely. In other words, the research literature has uncovered a problem, to which there should be a solution. The solution, within a majority of the research literature, is sought after by looking for *reasons* for variation in rates, in an implicit or explicit attempt to remedy the variations.

4.1.3. The first answer: patients matter

The majority of research, or what is understood as doxic representations within the research literature, is divided when answering this question: reasons for hospitalization are either connected to patient or facility specific factors (Carter & Porell 2003). Researchers analyzing patient specific factors generally focus on whether or not rates of hospitalization are associated with patient characteristics or patient demographics. For instance; if nursing home residents in California are hospitalized more frequently than residents in Florida, can this be explained by differences in the people living in California and Florida? In other words, are rates of hospitalization connected to characteristics or composition of patients?

This question can be further divided into several subsections. Some focus on general characteristics of patient demographics (such as age, gender, education and ethnicity) (Grabowski et al. 2008, Carter 2003a, Culler et al. 1998, Freiman & Murtaugh 1993, Murtaugh & Freiman 1995, Ouslander et al. 2010, Pappas & Hadden 1997). Some focus on the association between patient demographics and specific diagnosis (the prevalence of pneumonia in a geographical area or for those aged above 80 years, for instance) (Freiman & Murtaugh 1993, Fried & Mor 1997, Konetzka et al. 2008, Loeb et al. 2006, O'Malley et al. 2011). Yet others focus on the association between patient demographics and institutions' selection of population (Culler et al. 1998). Some studies have demonstrated a connection between the variation in socioeconomic background of residents and outcomes, including rates of hospitalization (Carter 2003a, Culler et al. 1998, Pappas & Hadden 1997). Others highlight the differences in structural conditions as important for patient demographics in nursing homes, especially costs of residency, and methods of financing (Pappas & Hadden 1997). Higher income per capita, for instance, has been shown to increase chances of hospitalization (Carter 2003a).

Somewhere between the realm of patient and facility specific factors lies the related topic of how specific conditions or diagnoses are *treated* differently, such as falls (Godden & Pollock 2001), bed sores (Konetzka et al. 2008), and dementia (Phelan et al. 2012). Dementia, for instance, is also found to be associated with increased risk of being hospitalized for potentially preventable conditions (Ibid.). This topic borders on the realm of facility specific factors, as one could argue that the independent variable is treatment methods rather than the occurrence of the diagnosis itself.

Even though resident level factors can contribute to a heterogeneous patient demographic and thus can explain some of the variations in rates of hospitalization, especially across large geographical areas, it has been argued that such explanation factors are far from sufficient, in addition to producing contradictory findings (Carter & Porell 2003). The main weakness in arguing exclusively for patient-specific factors as determining rates of hospitalization is that variation in rates of hospitalization occurs within smaller homogeneous geographical areas (Carter 2003a, Carter & Porell 2003). If variations in rates within smaller homogeneous areas, serving the same demographic, are similar to variations across larger areas, variation cannot be exclusively explained by demographic variation. Based on this important, in my opinion, nuance, some of the researchers have conveyed the need to change the perspective from looking exclusively at patient-specific factors, to incorporating facility-specific factors (Carter 2003a, Horn et al. 2005, Zimmerman et al. 2002, Harrington et al. 2000). For a large section of the research on hospitalization, the perspective has shifted from patient demographics to the attributes of institutions.

4.1.4. The second answer: institutions matter/ institutional matter

It has been suggested that up to 48 percent of all hospitalizations can be explained by socio-cultural, rather than medical factors (Cohen-Mansfield & Lipson 2006). Leaving the problematic term «socio-cultural factors» aside for now, which factors or conditions are relevant?

Financing/Ownership/Profit status: Generally it is argued that chain-affiliated nursing homes have a higher rate of hospitalization than non-chain affiliated nursing homes (Carter & Porell 2003, Zimmerman et al. 2002). Similarly, findings indicate that for- profit nursing homes hospitalize their residents more often than non-profit nursing homes (Anderson et al. 1998, Carter 2003a, Carter & Porell 2003, Konetzka et al. 2004, OIG 2013, McGregor et al. 2014, Zimmerman et al. 2002). A majority, but not all, of chain-affiliated homes are for-profit, hence the division. In different ways, financing has been shown to be associated with rates of hospitalizations (Anderson et al. 1998, Coleman & Berenson 2004, Grabowski et al. 2008, Konetzka et al. 2004, Mor et al. 2010a, Mor et al. 2010b). As many of the financing methods are specific to regions or countries, and therefore lack a general relevance, a detailed account will not be given[1]. In addition, the occurrence and form of «advance directives» or the equivalent seem to vary between countries and regions[2]; they are more formalized in North America than in Scandinavia, for instance. Few studies cover this topic directly, while they do find contradicting evidence when it comes to a connection with rates of hospitalization (Hutt et al. 2002), when the topic is addressed.

Nursing home size: In many of the research articles nursing home size is said to be more directly correlated to rates of hospitalization (Anderson et al. 1998, Barker et al. 1994, McGregor et al. 2014, OIG 2013); larger nursing homes hospitalize more often than smaller ones. Research articles that analyze a variety of facility specific factors and their respective effect on rates of hospitalization, of which there are several, usually highlight size as the factor with the highest correlation. However, such studies, as we shall see later, seldom analyze how the factors *influence each other*, as well as rates of hospitalization.

Nurse staffing patterns: The ways in which nursing home staff influence hospitalization has been covered extensively by the research literature (Anderson et al. 1998, Anderson et al. 2003, Carter 2003a, Carter 2003b, Decker 2006, Decker 2008, Dellefield 2000, Harrington et al. 2000, Intrator et al. 1999, Konetzka et al. 2008, Weech-Maldonado et al. 2004, Zimmerman et al. 2002). The literature typically focuses on a) whether or not an isolated professional category influences hospitalization or b) the composition of the different professional categories and what composition is optimal. The effect of the number of nurses employed on hospitalization is especially debated. Some state that increasing the number of *registered* nurses (RNs) decreases hospitalization (Anderson et al. 1998, Anderson et al. 2003, Carter 2003b, Carter & Porell 2005, Decker 2006, Decker 2008, McGregor et al. 2014) or «*deficiencies*» (Harrington et al. 2000), especially if the alternative is licensed practical nurses (LPNs), licensed vocational nurses (LVNs) or similar categories (Anderson

---

1   See Kayser-Jones´ groundbreaking ethnographic study (1990) for an in-depth analysis of systemic and everyday effects of for-profit ownership, regarding, among other issues, incentives connected to accountability.

2   While prevalent in many countries, advanced directives are not common in Norway. Even the most common form of «life testaments» are not widespread, nor are they legally binding (Schaffer 2007). International literature points to conflicting findings regarding the effect of advanced directives on the decision making process, arguing, for instance, that directives fail to properly guide nursing home staff in decisions (Lopez 2009, Terrell & Miller 2006).

et al. 1998, Carter 2003b, Dellefield 2000, Kayser-Jones et al. 1989). Others show contradicting or modifying evidence (Intrator et al. 1999, Konetzka et al. 2008, O'Malley et al. 2011). The relationship between the RN and the LPN/LVN and how the composition of these categories relates to hospitalization, have also been debated, perhaps because in some respect they overlap, and therefore are in a competitive relationship when it comes to influence in the nursing home. The administration at the nursing home has a strong incentive to employ LVNs rather than RNs, as they perform similar tasks, but are cheaper to employ (Anderson et al. 1998).

In general, the topic of staffing patterns is widely debated, but without, it has been argued, sufficient attention to how professional groups interact and how the institutional context as a whole can serve as a premise for decisions on hospitalization (Grabowski et al. 2008). Such a dearth has later been modified by the inclusion of other approaches (Chapter 4.1.5).

Physician staffing patterns: Based on the premise that avoidable hospitalizations exist, one would think that increased coverage of physicians decreases hospitalization. Some studies have found this association to have some merit (Intrator et al. 1999), indicating that more physician hours per resident per day are considered to decrease the chances of hospitalization. However, findings are not always conclusive on this point (Grabowski et al. 2008, Jensen et al. 2009, Miller & Weissert 2000), or might even be contradictory (Intrator et al. 2004). The findings on the effect on hospitalization of having an «on site physician» (as opposed to general practitioners employed on an hourly basis) are similarly inconclusive (Grabowski et al. 2008). Personal style, belief and differences in education, have also been pointed out as influencing variations between physicians when it comes to decisions on hospitalization (Cohen-Mansfield & Lipson 2006), but are not analyzed explicitly within the majority of research.

Turnover/job satisfaction: The literature on this topic is extensive, covering level of turnover for different professions (administrators, physicians, RNs, and LPNs), number of tenured staff versus temporary staff, as well as how these different factors affect outcomes for patients. High turnover rates are associated with negative outcomes for patients, including elevated rates of hospitalization (Collier & Harrington 2008, Zimmerman et al. 2002). Castle has argued that there is a connection between quality of care and turnover, and likewise between turnover and job satisfaction, making the latter an important instrument for improving quality of care (Castle 2001a, 2001b, 2005, & Castle et al. 2007). Rates of turnover have received much attention in the research literature, as they can be exceptionally high in nursing homes in the United States, often exceeding 75 percent, sometimes reaching as high as 400 percent (Banaaszak-Holl & Hines 1996). However, as we will see later, such is not the case for our nursing homes.

To summarize, a large portion of the literature has drifted away from only focusing on characteristics and composition of patients as explanations for varying institutional practices, to including factors related to institutions and policy. Some argue explicitly for the need to study facility level factors or socio-cultural aspects for a balanced and thorough understanding of the mechanisms leading to hospitalization (Carter 2003a, Harrington et al. 2000, Horn et al. 2005, Zimmerman et al. 2002). This need has been met by a segment of the research literature applying alternative approaches and designs.

4.1.5. The third answer: process and practice

Another segment of the research literature can be isolated and treated as distinctively separate from the majority of research based on differences in design and approaches: research with the overall common denominator of being «qualitative». «Qualitative research» is a vague and wide-ranging term, as is the application of the term for research on hospitalization from nursing homes, most notably in two recent literature reviews (Arendts et al. 2013, Laging et al. 2015), including research using observation, interviews, focus groups and questionnaires as primary methodological approaches. This segment of the research literature is distinguishable from other segments not only by approach, but also by time of publication. They are, on average, more recent and are, consequently, able to draw on experiences and findings from others. This segment can be labelled as the heterodoxa to the doxa of the research literature by applying different approaches and designs on a similar topic, while being in a minority and, as we shall see, fragmented.

In the most recent review (Laging et al. 2015), which included findings from the former (where, for some reason, observational studies were excluded, Arendts et al. 2013: 826), the qualitative research literature on hospitalization from nursing homes is described as varied and having a «(...) *lack of consensus regarding the role of the nursing home when a resident's health deteriorates*»

(Laging et al. 2015: 1). Upon further analysis of the respective studies one by one, such a sentiment is accentuated, in addition to revealing that many studies do not, at least explicitly, actually cover the topic of hospitalization from nursing homes. Five of 17 included studies cover the topic of «*end-of life*» or «*palliative care*» exclusively, thus excluding acute illness in residents not considered to be dying. Another five of 17 included studies exclusively address transfers to emergency wards as opposed to hospitals. Finally, eight of the included studies exclusively analyze *perceptions of transfers* (to emergency wards, hospitals or both), as opposed to the transfers themselves, based on retrospective accounts and interpretations from informants. Several other included studies analyzed perceptions of transfers, but also included other sources of data.

The included qualitative research is somewhat more varied regarding country of origin than the majority of research, although still predominantly from North America (two from Norway, four from Australia, four from Canada and seven from the United States). The research is not as varied regarding applied methodological approach: a large majority (14) utilize interviews and focus groups (either in isolation or in combination) as their main approach, while the remaining three use observation and/or participant observation as their main approach (all of which also used interviews). Of the three, two applied a longitudinal or prospective design (Kayser-Jones et al. 1989 and McCloskey 2011), while Lopez (2009) interviewed participants in the decision-making process retrospectively.

The literature is relevant for our purposes as all studies have a common trait in covering the topic of how and why residents of nursing homes are transferred from the nursing home in cases of acute illness or approaching death, either explicitly or implicitly. Even though research varies in its specific area of interest (dying residents versus all residents, hospitals versus emergency wards, perceptions of practice versus conducted practice, for instance) the respective emphasis on influential factors for transfers are strikingly similar. Recurrent themes and emphases can be synthesized into five areas: four specific - the role of nurses, physicians, family and availability of treatment options, and one conceptual - a focus on the decision-making process.

The role of nurses and/or registered nurses in decisions to transfer residents out of the nursing home is given substantial emphasis in the research literature, pointing to their explicit or implicit influence on most decisions. Such an emphasis is a contrast to other segments of the research literature, in which the role of the physician is primary: *«Despite this central role, most studies of transfer decision-making focus on the physician»* (Bottrell et al. 2001). It would seem that when changing the perspective from the decision itself, or the outcome of a decision, to what leads to the decision, nurses are increasingly at center stage. The focus on the significance of nurses might also be attributed to the fact that most studies are *about* nurses[3] and many are carried out *by* nurses[4]. Nurses or registered nurses, it is argued, are central in decision-making about residents in general (Arendts & Howard 2010, Bottrell et al. 2001, Carusone et al. 2006a, Kayser-Jones et al. 1989, Mitchell et al. 2011, Shanley et al. 2011, Shidler 1998), because of formal responsibility and authority (McCloskey 2011), or through indirect or subtle influences over others (Jablonski et al. 2007, Lopez 2009). Although most studies highlight the benevolent role of the nurse, torn between opposing interests, the nurse can, in some instances, also influence decisions based on convenience or because of pressure from others, arguments rarely found in the other segments of the research literature:

> *«In several cases, the nursing staff asked physicians to transfer patients who required heavy nursing care. These residents were seen as difficult to care for, and in some cases the administration wanted them moved because of fear of receiving a citation from state inspectors.»* (Kayser-Jones et al. 1989)

While the general emphasis is directed towards the influence of nurses and registered nurses, and the importance of sound coverage of these groups, some of the studies also point to composition of staff, or skill-mix, as influential in the decision process (Arendts & Howard 2010, Shanley et al. 2011). Lopez (2009) also emphasizes the difficulty for the nurse of being torn between the wishes of families, physicians, residents and their perceptions of residents' best interests, potentially diminishing the role of nurses in the decision process. Few studies incorporate the role of assistants in analysis of the decision process, making Phillips' (et al. 2006) discussion of assistants' vague and shifting influence an important contribution.

---

3   Of the 14 studies utilizing interviews and/or focus groups (Laging et al. 2015), 11 did so with nurses, either exclusively (seven studies) or in combination with administrators and/or assistants (four studies). The remaining three studies interviewed administrators exclusively.

4   Seven of the 17 studies are first authored by registered nurses (Laging et al. 2015), five by other professional groups. The remaining five did not disclose professional background of first author.

The role of the physician is less emphasized than that of the nurse in this part of the literature. The physician is typically presented as having varied influence on transfer decisions when discussed (Laging et al. 2015). Studies point out that a lack of access to physicians influences (in the sense of increasing) rates of hospitalization (Jablonski et al. 2007, McCloskey 2011, Phillips et al. 2006), either in general, or at times when the physician in not physically present at the nursing homes (Mitchell et al. 2011). Others emphasize challenges in communication between physicians and nurses (and families) as potentially influencing decisions of transfer (Phillips et al. 2006). The first and, in several ways, most groundbreaking study within this part of the literature (Kayser-Jones et al. 1989) highlights physicians' convenience as significant for transfers. It is argued that physicians in nursing homes are not adequately compensated for their work (at least not to the degree they are outside the nursing home) and therefore are de-incentivized to treat residents especially on multiple occasions (Ibid.). In general, physicians are not presented as having the sole, or in some instances even major, responsibility and/or influence over decisions of transfer, and are, in many cases, not present. When present, physicians are presented as being receptive of being manipulated by caring staff: again an area not covered by other segments of the literature.

The largest difference of attributed emphasis on decisions of transfer between this and other parts of the literature revolves around the role of the family of residents. Potential pressure from family to transfer or not to transfer residents (more often the former) is accentuated in several studies and is noticeably missing from other segments of the literature. Family of residents is pointed out to be generally influential, through interaction with physicians, nurses or both (Arendts & Howard 2010, Bottrell et al. 2001, Hutt et al. 2011, Jablonski et al. 2007, Kayser-Jones et al. 1989, Lamb et al. 2011, Phillips et al. 2006, Shanley et al. 2011): or in specific cases when the resident's preferences were unknown (Lopez 2009). Staff in nursing homes experience pressure from family, it is generally argued, while the *effect* of pressure varies, depending on the study.

The topic of treatment options or services is also covered in other segments of the literature, but is approached somewhat differently in the qualitative literature. Rather than exclusively addressing the *availability* of treatment options (such as intravenous therapy), the literature highlights *variation in utilization* of available treatment options (Jablonski et al. 2007,

Kayser-Jones et al. 1989). In addition, the relationship between availability, utilization of and having adequately trained staff, is pointed out as influential for decisions on hospitalization (Carusone et al. 2006a & 2006b). Even so, treatment options are not attributed the same amount of significance as the other aspects mentioned.

As evident in the review of these four areas highlighted by the qualitative research, the general emphasis for most studies, regardless of approach and attributed significance, is on the decision-making process leading to transfers, as opposed to outcome of transfers. It would appear that when such a shift in focus is made; that is from being exclusively directed towards the patient or towards characteristics of the institutions, nurses and families are attributed increased significance. As such, the perspective is moved from facility specific factors to processual dynamics. Nonetheless, not all areas of the decision-making process are extensively covered by this part of the literature, most notably missing being *potential hospitalizations*.

The qualitative studies provide insight into aspects not covered by other parts of the literature. Still, these studies, although addressing additional or supplementary areas of interest, remain limited. Much has been confirmed since the first groundbreaking study of Kayser-Jones (et al. 1989), but little has been added: «*Interestingly, the factors identified in the contemporary studies are the same as those found by Kayser-Jones et al. in 1989, suggesting that little has changed as far as the factors that influence NH staff decision-making over the past 25 years*» (Laging et al. 2015: 9). Perhaps also little has changed in adding to, nuancing and theorizing the findings from 1989. While the qualitative literature illuminates an area of study potentially significant for practice in nursing homes, including that of hospitalization (how and by whom decisions are made), it does not treat the fundamental question of how decisions are developed, nor of how they are founded, including that of structural influences. The literature does not raise the question from where such practices are generated.

4.2. Literature on hospitalization – Norway

The literature on nursing homes in Norway is fairly rich in size and scope. Few, however, address the topic of hospitalization from nursing homes directly, as does the research literature from other Scandinavian countries.

A few studies do, nonetheless, stand out, briefly described in Chapter 2.3. As mentioned, these studies do not attempt an in-depth and/or wide-ranging analysis of explanations for overall and variations of rates of hospitalization. Some findings and suggestions for further studies should still be mentioned.

Two of the previously cited studies analyze the influence of institutional conditions for the occurrence and variation of rates of hospitalization, Graverholt by analyzing the significance of size, location, ownership and types of beds on rates of hospitalization (et al. 2013) and Krüger by including size, types of beds and physician coverage (et al. 2011). Graverholt found a significant correlation between nursing home size and rate of hospitalization (smaller nursing homes hospitalize more often than larger) and for percentage of short-term beds (more short-term beds, more hospitalization). Note that size has the opposite effect of what has been argued for in a majority of the international literature. Krüger's study found a similar correlation for percentage of short-term beds (et al. 2011), a finding that, given the general function of short-term beds, is not surprising. Location of nursing homes and ownership status produced no effects (Graverholt et al. 2013). The authors argue for a more uniform practice based on their findings (Ibid.). In Krüger's study, hospitalization rates were also found to be associated with physician coverage (more physician coverage, more hospitalization), for nursing homes with short-term beds (et al. 2011, see also Steen et al. 2009). This is a somewhat contradictory finding to that of Graverholt, arguing that smaller nursing homes (who hospitalize more than larger) have less physician coverage than larger (Graverholt et al. 2013).

Although these studies do not attempt a wide-ranging analysis of the *association* between potentially relevant factors, or the everyday practices in nursing homes, Graverholt in particular raises some pertinent questions for further discussions. The high figure for overall rates of hospitalization is questioned as being symptomatic of the general characteristics of residents in Norwegian nursing homes - old and frail - or of cultural particularities surrounding the notion of what the nursing home is and should be.

Regardless of the reasons for overall rates of hospitalization, *the variation* in rates of hospitalization between institutions cannot be explained by the *general* characteristics of residents. One could make the argument that Norway, compared to many other countries, has a relatively homogeneous population of elderly, especially when it comes to ethnicity and social class. Such an argument is echoed in Graverholt's study, stating that «(...) *we anticipate that the characteristics of the nursing home population are distributed evenly across the nursing homes studied.*» (Graverholt et al. 2013: 5). Such an apparent universality does not explain variation, but rather points to the improbability of resident demographics being a decisive factor in explaining *differences* in rates of hospitalization. Thus, variation remains largely unexplained, a point also alluded to by Graverholt, stating that differences in «*professional cultures*» (labelled *practice* here) and «*organizational factors*», not included in their study, might be significant in explaining such a perplexing variation. The hypothesis is supported, it is argued, firstly by the relative stability of variation between institutions over a two-year period. Secondly, it is theorized that «(...) *the characteristics we have studied may represent proxies or markers of other characteristics closer to the problem, like composition of staffing, management and culture*» (Graverholt et al. 2013: 5). Although the very existence of variation does in itself not necessarily constitute a «problem», the hypothesis is interesting and will be explored in this book.

To summarize: there are distinct similarities in design and approach between the respective segments of the Norwegian and international literature, even though the Norwegian literature is small in size and on average relies on a smaller population sample. As such, the Norwegian research literature referenced follows the pattern of the international research literature of being grounded in different research traditions that do not overlap, in which one tradition appears to represent a dominant position; the doxa within the field of research. The quantitatively oriented studies, for instance, seem to share the international literature's emphasis on variation as empirically surprising and/or normatively problematic. Nursing homes should hospitalize similarly, it is implied.

In sum, the international, and to some degree the national, literature on hospitalization from nursing homes is rich in size and analyzes a large variation of relevant factors connected to rates of hospitalization. It is somewhat varied when it comes to methodological approaches and research designs, although qualitative studies are in a minority, especially for observational studies looking beyond *perceptions* of the object of study. I will argue that the study of hospitalizations from nursing homes could be strengthened by added emphasis on areas not extensively covered by the research literature.

4.3. Black holes: areas of improvement

Based primarily on the prevalent study design and approach, leading to what can be described as doxic representations, the research literature on hospitalization from nursing homes is dominated by certain perspectives and emphases. A similar argument was made in a thought-provoking theoretical review of research on nursing home residents in emergency departments (McCloskey & Hoonaard 2007), which argued that «(…) *power derived from medical knowledge is used by emergency department personnel to construct nursing home residents as problematic»* (186). It is further argued that the research literature is severely limited regarding the effects of transfers on nursing homes (as opposed to the emergency wards), events in nursing homes leading to transfers and accounts provided by nursing homes staff or residents (Ibid.). Research, it is argued, is focused on physicians and the effects of transfers on emergency departments, primarily driven or implemented by physicians, and executed by way of a uniform and simplistic design: retrospective record reviews being traced back from the end-point, the emergency ward (Ibid.). While it is easy to agree with the general arguments made by McCloskey & Hoonaard regarding the uniformity of research focus and design as well as the tendency in a majority of research literature to *assume* that many hospitalizations are inappropriate, I will attempt to nuance two major arguments made. McCloskey & Hoonard argue that the division between «*the medical model»* (hospitals) and the nursing homes' «*system of care»* is distinct and non-transgressional, characterized by the execution of power by one over the other. The one-sided emphasis in the research literature is seen as a consequence of such a display of power. Rather than seeing the systems as strictly opposed and as dominant/dominated, I will suggest that the medical model should be viewed as adopted and integrated *into* nursing homes, in a concrete *and* in a conceptual sense. Such a position is more in accordance with the notion of doxa than Foucault's notion of «power», adopted by the cited researchers. A medical model is adopted into nursing homes, it will be argued, *as a medically oriented research tradition incorporated into nursing or care sciences.* In contrast to McCloskey & Hoonard's findings, a substantial part of the research literature is executed by and covers perspectives from nurses (and not simply physicians), while their perspectives, methodological approaches and (lack of) theoretical foundation remain cemented in a rather strict medically-oriented tradition.

I will argue that sufficient emphasis has not been placed on a) *potential* hospitalizations, b) the interplay between potential relevant factors, and c) everyday practice in the nursing home. These areas are related, and all share the characteristic of being areas to which it is difficult for the researcher to gain immediate access. The areas of interplay between factors and everyday practices are covered to some extent by the research literature: particularly by the qualitative research, but not extensively enough given what is in question. Certain aspects of the study of nursing homes, most notably a study of the generation of practice (rather than perceptions of practice), is still missing from the increasingly completed puzzle.

4.3.1. Potential hospitalizations

Research about the decision making process relating to hospitalization is substantial in terms of the number of articles addressing the topic, both in the qualitative literature and other segments (Brooks et al. 1994, Cohen-Mansfield et al. 2003a, Cohen-Mansfield et al. 2003b, Cohen-Mansfield & Lipson 2006, Flacker et al. 2001). This research, however, rarely incorporates analyses of decisions *not* resulting in a hospitalization. Research tends to analyze *actual* hospitalizations, more often than not, retrospectively. Within the majority of research, whose mission it is, as argued, to understand variations in rates of hospitalization, *potential hospitalizations* (that is, hospitalizations that do not occur, but could occur at other institutions) are completely missing, thus leaving out half the picture (see Boockvar et al. 2005 for an exception).

This apparent paradox, that studies on variations do not incorporate that which is varied, has been addressed by Cohen-Mansfield, arguing that the initial process must be identified and understood for a complete analysis of the decision making process (Cohen-Mansfield et al. 2003a). By excluding potential hospitalizations, then, a potential significant source for the analysis of variation is missing. In general, I will argue that the proclivity for retrospective (rather than longitudinal) designs based on statistical (rather than observational) analysis, leaves a majority of the research literature blind to the potential significance of a focus on potential hospitalization for the analysis of *variation of practices* between nursing homes.

4.3.2. The interplay between conditions

As seen, an emphasis on the organizational characteristics, as a supplement to patient characteristics, is warranted, as is an emphasis on the decision-making process as a supplement to organizational characteristics. Even though the different segments of the research literature analyze the influence of various factors on rates of hospitalizations, most of the research literature overlooks the potential *connections between* the various factors, both within and between each segment. Even though some research articles focus on several factors and their respective significance for hospitalization, the significance remains just that, *respective*. As pointed out in one of the literature reviews (Grabowski et al. 2008), studies evaluate the importance of *overall* staffing levels, and the importance of *composition* of staff, but do not evaluate how, for example, these are connected. In other words, a majority of research articles treat factors as being relevant to hospitalization, but as working *independently* from each other. While some researchers, for example, analyze the interplay between financing, ownership, staffing levels and hospitalization, many researchers fail to grasp such a dynamic. Rather, the objective seems to be to search for single variables as answers, rather than analyzing variations and connections of factors.

Exceptions are to be found within each segment of the literature. The work of McGregor et al. (2010 & 2014) on continuity of physician care and transfers to emergency departments from nursing homes is a rare example[5] of retrospective/quantitative design where researchers incorporate both the interdependence of various factors for hospitalizations and analyze relevant factors in terms of *how* care is provided, rather than only focusing on *how much* and *by whom*. The role of the physician is nuanced in this research, by demonstrating how *continuity* of physician care matters, measured both by number of patients per physician and how «*timely attendants are*», and is seen as relational to other institutional characteristics (McGregor et al. 2010, McGregor et al. 2014). In a study of decisions on transfers to emergency departments, Jablonski (et al. 2007) makes a similar contribution to the research literature by nuancing the relative and changing influence of families, physicians and nurses, depending, among other factors, on the composition of those involved.

---

5   See also Zimmerman (et al. 2002).

The qualitative literature in general is less preoccupied with isolating specific factors of influence on hospitalizations (in an attempt to find *the solution*), but does still, for the most part, fail to address influencing factors *outside* of the specific decisions that are made, being institutional or structural. The potential influence of the overall structural framework, particularly in the form of legislation, regulations and guidelines, is noticeably missing from the qualitative and parts of the quantitative literature (emphasizing financial, rather than regulatory influences), perhaps because these tend to be context-specific.

The need to analyze the connection between relevant factors is not only a question of epistemology and methodological approach (being quantitative or qualitative), but is also related to the general attributes of nursing homes, to what nursing homes «are». «*Because few nursing facilities tend to differ from others on only one attribute at a time, there is difficulty in substantively gauging the cumulative impact of facility-level factors in our empirical findings*» (Carter & Porell 2003: 185). Analyzing how factors or conditions work together cumulatively within and between nursing homes is, in other words, a challenging scientific exercise. It still remains *an important* scientific exercise, as a more wide-ranging approach will be better suited to analyzing the potentially significant relationships between relevant factors on different levels. In doing so, analyses can contribute to an understanding of the *causes* for what appears in most studies as statistical significance (as opposed to simply stating a significance). As will be discussed, other factors than those immediately apparent can cause statistical significance, in the form for instance of sporadic and spurious effects. The statistical significance of size of nursing homes, as demonstrated by several studies, could for some institutions be explained by factors *connected to size*, rather than size itself, and/or by more or less coincidental occurrences such as one or two residents at small nursing homes.

4.3.3. The practice of day-to-day care

In the majority of the research literature, representing the research doxa, the general topic of the interaction between staff and patients is not covered. Little emphasis is placed on the *content* of care, as opposed to the *organization* of care. Consequently, how the practice of day-to-day care can explain differences between institutions is to a large degree overlooked. In most of the literature, then, care is not studied as a *process*[6] (or as the *modus operandi*, (Bourdieu 2012: 18-19)), but rather as a fixed entity, easily measured (as the *opus operatum*, Ibid.). The interaction between staff and residents is either not studied or presented as being a fixed, measurable entity, independent of time. There is little or no emphasis on the *content* of the interaction between and among caring staff, physicians and residents. Consequently, how the practice of day-to-day care can influence decisions on hospitalization, and how it can explain differences between institutions, is to a large degree overlooked. This is particularly puzzling when taking into account the large number of residents with Alzheimer´s disease in nursing homes (Carter & Porell 2005) making communication between resident and staff challenging at best. In addition, the high prevalence of falls in nursing homes (Rubenstein et al. 1996, Spector et al. 2007), which make ad-hoc preventive measures of different kinds an important part of everyday life, further illustrates the need for analyses of everyday life in nursing homes.

This area of research marks the greatest contribution of the qualitative research literature, by focusing on decisions made in nursing homes by those involved. Although the segment represents a much-needed supplement to the existing knowledge bank, it also has its limitations. Only a few studies within this segment of the literature actually study the process of decisions, while most analyze agents' *perceptions of the process*. Additionally, a majority of the qualitative literature fails to analyze how the process of decisions can be shaped or influenced by contextual and structural elements, resulting in a presentation of agents who exhibit an absolute rationalism (although emotionally involved) on an individual or group (nurse, family or physician) level.

The study of everyday practice can, in addition to its intrinsic value to the understanding of decisions and variation of decisions, also uncover contradictions to «rules» (being concrete or conceptual). The «rule» of physicians' presence in nursing homes being a fixed entity at Norwegian nursing homes (Graverholt et al. 2013) is, for instance, a rule which can be bent and interpreted differently.

---

6   An exception to this tendency is a subtheme dealing with communication between NHs and hospitals/ emergency wards (Brooks et al. 1994, Cheng et al. 2006, Coleman 2003, Coleman & Berenson 2004, Cwinn et al. 2009, Parry et al. 2003). Within this subtheme, the focus is on processes influencing hospitalizations, rather than specific factors.

4.3.4. Summary

The research literature, which can be said to be composed of a dominant and an opposing research discourse, is, in my opinion, representative of a doxa that results in certain limitations. These limitations - that which remains undiscussed – can be seen as relating to the chosen research designs and approaches, which limit the gaze with which nursing homes are studied.

As will be argued, including those who are not hospitalized (but could have been) is an important approach to the analysis of variation between nursing homes. Furthermore, a focus on potential hospitalizations leaves the researcher capable of analyzing how factors can be interrelated (Chapter 5) and more or less dependent on everyday practice in nursing homes (Chapter 9). The analysis of the interrelatedness of structural and institutional conditions for the practice of hospitalization (Chapter 5), meanwhile, further contributes to an understanding of *variation* between nursing homes, while the analysis of everyday practice in nursing homes, (Chapter 9), can explain how such variations are generated and implemented. In general, the research literature tends to explain practices of hospitalization either as relating causally to specific factors functioning outside the everyday practice of agents' involvement or as dependent on the rationale of agents making decisions independently of institutional or structural conditions.

What matters? A small chapter about complexity

As argued in Chapter 4, a significant segment of the research literature studying hospitalizations from nursing homes treats influencing factors as having an intrinsic value and, therefore, an inherent effect on hospitalization, more or less irrespective of the specific context of the respective nursing homes. The effect of a factor is typically presented as being universal, that is as being valid for most or all nursing homes within a given sample, rather than being connected to the context of individual or samples of nursing homes. Size of institution, for instance, is presented as influencing rates of hospitalization in a more or less deterministic way, without accounting for other factors *relating* to size or the contextual features.

I will argue for the need to understand how relevant factors interplay inside, and not just across, the walls of the institutions. The actual decisions made at the institutions are dependent on many, related considerations, not easily accessible to the researcher, or even to the practitioner herself, and not necessarily transferable from one nursing home or jurisdiction to the next. Often many of these factors interact dynamically to influence the decision-making process, making it more complex and more challenging to analyze. Nursing homes «(…) *like the rest of the healthcare system, are complex adaptive institutions, and it is likely that these apparently contradictory associations may be explained by unmeasured factors producing confounding effects*» (McGregor et al. 2014: 9).

Furthermore, a broad-ranging analysis of factors influencing the decision-making process can be a key to understanding the variations in rates of hospitalization, as it may unveil how different factors can be relevant in different places at different times, thus perhaps explaining *variations* in rates including those within smaller geographical areas.

To make sense and make progress in a potentially extensive, complicated and multi-faceted area, only a selection of the many potentially relevant factors at play in nursing homes are included. The factors included are based on those given the most emphasis in the different segments of the literature presented, also including issues not covered extensively by the literature, but potentially of significance. Based on these considerations, an analytical division has been constructed between a) the overall structural framework potentially influencing decisions on hospitalizations (national legislation, for instance), and b) conditional influences related to the characteristics of the respective institutions and/or staff. These factors will be analyzed in relation to what extent they *determine practice* in nursing homes, and to what degree nursing homes are left with opportunities, choice and dependence contributing to variation.

5.1. The structure

«Structure» and «context» can be, and have been, understood and referred to in several, not necessarily compatible ways. Here, the structural framework will be referred to as the overall, generic context, the macro-level, to which all nursing homes must relate. These elements, most notably national (or regional, depending on the country) policies, laws and regulations, and the general financial framework and mechanisms affecting both the nursing home industry and the daily operation of specific institutions, are elements to which all nursing homes must adhere, as is their very nature. These two aspects of the structural framework will be treated superficially in the following; primarily addressing to what degree they influence and/or determine the everyday practices in nursing homes. I will argue that within a shared context, which for our case is primarily a national context, nursing homes relate similarly to the structural framework. This provides nursing homes with a set of non-specific premises creating a space in which practice can be generated.

Policies, legislation and regulations, for example, provide a universal framework for nursing homes within a given area, to which they must relate *similarly*. The structural framework, then, is meant to create «an even playing field», if not equality.

In the case of Norway, governance, responsibility and accountability are placed primarily within the domain of the respective municipalities. As such, the model of governance in Norway can facilitate differences *between* municipalities, but not necessarily (certainly not automatically) *within* them. In addition to placing a large bulk of the responsibility for implementing national policies locally, both national and municipal policies can be described as being relatively non-specific. Policies and regulations, in other words, do not micro-manage the everyday operations of nursing homes. The daily operations of nursing homes cannot be deduced or traced back to the policies and regulations to which they relate. More specifically, national and municipal policies and regulations do not speak explicitly of hospitalizations[1], although specifying that residents (or family of residents) have the legal right to refuse treatment at end-of-life. Nursing homes are not required to follow or even be advised on practices relating to hospitalizations, either in principle or with regards to specific treatments or diagnoses. Policies and regulations can still be said to be indirectly influential for practices relating to hospitalizations in the sense of providing a generic framework, especially concerning staffing patterns, compositions of residents of nursing homes and the financial operations of nursing homes. Nursing homes must relate similarly to these factors, while their specific implementation, which can take different forms, can affect how decisions of hospitalization are made. The implementation of the previously mentioned Coordination Reform – perhaps the most explicitly relevant form of governmental policy for nursing homes' practices of hospitalization (and thus an exception to the general argument of their non-specific form) - can serve as a brief example of the relative autonomy of local interpretation, implementation and strategy connected to their structural framework. In the first stages of local implementation, nursing homes from our sample adjusted differently and at different times to the reform. Some of the nursing homes related explicitly to the new reform, by discussing its consequences and adjusting certain practices, while others did not, taking a position along the line of «waiting

---

1 The scope and content of regulations and guidelines specifically on practices of hospitalization have caught the attention of some research (see Chapter 4). However, such regulations and guidelines tend to be context-specific and not transferable to a Norwegian setting. *The effect* of regulations and guidelines, however, might be transferable and translatable to a Norwegian context. Studies on this area point to contrary findings: in one study, the implementation of guidelines for the treatment of pneumonia did not affect rates of hospitalization, primarily as *«secular pressure»* -in part in the form of families of residents- undermined the guidelines (Hutt et al. 2011); while another study found that the implementation of a *«clinical pathway»* reduced hospitalizations for pneumonia (and similar ailments) by 12 percent, without decreasing quality of life of those hospitalized (Loeb et al. 2006).

to see what would transpire». Most administrators stated the reform's significance, while not being quite certain of *how* it was significant.

From the perspective of our nursing homes, as will be discussed later (see Chapter 9.1), policies, laws and regulations, which can be merged into a concept of «rules» to which nursing homes must adhere, provide (relatively unspecific) premises from which nursing homes create independent sets of routines, forming the basis of everyday life.

Financial mechanisms, including models of payment for residents, public reimbursement schemes and national or regional regulations concerning the financial operations of nursing homes, can be said to be a part of the structural framework for nursing homes on several, related levels. Nursing homes might, for instance, be incentivized to seek treatment elsewhere for their residents if reimbursement schemes are unfavorable for treatment in-house, as pointed out in a study of nursing home directors (Bottrell et al. 2001). For similar reasons, emergency departments might be incentivized to return residents to nursing homes (McCloskey & Hoonaard 2007). As already discussed in Chapter 2, the general financial framework for nursing homes in Norway is relatively universal, for instance when it comes to revenue per bed. Historically, reimbursement schemes do not appear to have been significantly influential for decisions on hospitalization for Norwegian nursing homes, although this might be changing in light of the Coordination Reform. There are, however, variations *between municipalities*, particularly relating to total expenditure on nursing homes, connected to the general financial well-being of the respective municipalities. The general financial well-being of the respective municipalities, can, in other words, contribute to differences between nursing homes in different municipalities. Within municipalities, however, financial mechanisms, understood broadly, could be said to be similar to national policies and regulations in the sense that nursing homes relate to them on more or less equal terms.

However, certain aspects of the financial framework provided, as for national policies and regulations, leave room for local and varying interpretation, and consequently also for variation in practices. Nursing homes can *choose*, for instance, to relate differently to the dilemmas of filling vacancies. As mentioned, nursing homes, whether they answer to a municipal or corporate entity, are given relative independence by the municipality to allocate expenditures, for instance when it comes to total expenditures on salary for caring staff (although the specific wages are heavily regulated in Norway, compared to other countries). At one of our nursing homes, for instance, all vacancies except planned holidays were routinely not covered on the first day. For all vacancies caused by illness, in other words, the respective units had to suffice with one less staff than they were supposed to have. The regulatory framework and overview from the municipality do not cover potential sanctions for such a practice; in other words the institution was not accountable as they did not register or report the specific details of expenses for «salary».

The independent financial choices nursing home institutions can and, to a certain extent, have to make, are also evident with regard to equipment and food. A majority of nursing homes in our municipality, especially public ones, have, in an attempt to save revenue, outsourced production of warm meals to larger kitchens, located at other nursing homes. While such a financial effect can be debated, private nursing homes have autonomy in deciding whether they should provide warm meals themselves or not, as they also decide on using other sources of food. Public nursing homes have less autonomy in this matter; only a few larger institutions prepare their own meals. Provider agreements with various sources of goods follow a similar pattern; public nursing homes adhere to the municipal provider agreements, while the private sector can choose to, or not.

Both of the examples of filling vacancies (for all nursing homes) and ordering of goods (particularly for private nursing homes) point to *a potential* for local variation arising from the structural framework to which all nursing homes must relate. Nursing homes within the same area adapt differently – some choose to make their own warm meals, some choose to have registered nurses on-site at night-time, while some choose to buy more expensive diapers - thus facilitating different outcomes within a reasonably similar framework. But there is more at play than simply relating to each one of these choices independently; choosing more expensive diapers might influence financial flexibility in other matters, such as production of food, filling vacancies or treatment options.

In general, the structural framework, provides nursing homes with comparable premises, but also a substantial element of autonomy and choice. As such, the structural framework does not *create* differences between institutions, but rather *facilitates the possibility of variation. The possibility of variation* is accentuated by the local, more concrete context to which nursing homes relate *differently*.

5.2. The local

Institutional specific factors, as described beneath, include a variety of factors to which nursing homes must relate or by which they are influenced. For some of the factors, particularly size and physical layout, nursing homes have little room for influence or choice. Even so, nursing homes do differ in size and physical layout, have to relate and adapt given their size and layout, and are influenced on several levels by the respective characteristics of their size and layout. For other factors, such as staffing patterns and treatment options, nursing homes can influence the respective characteristics. Nursing homes can choose to have more registered nurses on rotation than the minimum or the average, and they can choose to offer intravenous treatment. The few included factors in the following, are included based on their varying significance for the development of sets of practices in nursing homes, including decisions on hospitalizations.

Nursing home size varies, within and outside our sample, nationally and internationally. While nursing homes cannot easily change size, either physically or in number of residents, size still matters. Size matters on several different, often related levels. The organization and autonomy of units, physician employment, physical layout, physical atmosphere (home-like or hospital-like), forms and size of organized activities (having an activity center, for instance), level of sick leave, size and influence of administration, degree of hierarchy between professional positions, among others, are all influenced in some way by size. Size, in itself, does not determine practices, but can influence them, *through* other relevant factors.

Nursing homes vary greatly in *physical layout*: in how they look, outside and inside their walls. Some nursing homes are new, some are old, and most are illustrative of the architectural preferences of the period in which they were built. The physical appearance of the interior of nursing homes varies with regard to the physical placement of units vis-à-vis each other and vis-à-vis common areas, entry point and administration; the ways in which units are shaped; and the placement (and sometimes existence) of common areas, activity centers and entry points. Units, meanwhile, vary between nursing homes in size, but also layout, including, but not exclusively, length and width of corridors; placement of rooms with regard to corridors, common rooms, kitchens and elevators; size and functionality of residents' rooms; and size and availability of common rooms. Generally, units in nursing homes are fairly similar within nursing homes when it comes to physical layout, but vary greatly between nursing homes. Differences between nursing homes include not only the physical appearance of rooms, but also decorations, and, relating to the latter, the more subtle atmosphere or ambience. Nursing homes can change the overall appearance of their hallways and rooms only to a limited degree, but can to a large degree manipulate decorations and atmosphere. As such, the physical look and «feel» of nursing homes *can* and *does* vary. Furthermore, physical layout and atmosphere is vitally important; it is where residents live and staff work. Physical layout and atmosphere also relate to several other factors; most notably size and ownership of nursing homes, organization and autonomy of units and staffing patterns. Lastly, as we will return to, physical layout is, *through its complex and potentially different relationship to other factors*, also influential for the development of practices in nursing homes, including decisions on hospitalization.

Regarding *composition of residents*, nursing homes in Norway have, as mentioned, little influence. Nursing homes can present requests to the respective municipal bodies, influencing the intake of a specific resident, and thereby influence the total level of acuity at a nursing home. If, for instance, a small nursing home has a proportionately high number of bedridden residents, they can request a more mobile resident. There are no guarantees, however, that these requests will be followed. The management of our six nursing homes, whether institutional leaders (for small nursing homes), or middle management or unit leaders (for large nursing homes), had very similar approaches towards distributing residents as evenly as possible among their respective units (based on the residents' assumed «caring needs»), while having different approaches towards their involvement and co-operation with the municipal agents. Some did not present requests at all, either because they did not see it as their job or because previous experience indicated that it would be futile, while some were very active in issuing requests, and saw it as a vital part of their jobs. The general lack of influence over patient composition does not by itself imply that variations in patient demographics will occur between nursing homes. And, as discussed previously, concluding on these matters, especially acuity level, is difficult and problematic relating both to access and size of sample. Still, it is safe to assume that the composition of residents, within our sample and in our municipality in general, is relatively similar. Nursing homes within our municipality cater to a relatively homogeneous population, making the differences between nursing homes seemingly less than in other countries. This assumption is supported by the data on resident characteristics, as presented earlier. Although different from nursing home residents of a previous sample (see Chapter 8.2.1), our sample is strikingly homogeneous when it comes to all categories included: age, level of dementia and ADLs. The population at our nursing homes does not seem to vary considerably.

Staffing patterns, including number and composition of caring staff in nursing homes, relate to the national and/or municipal structural framework, which provides guidelines for staffing, for instance having a registered nurse on duty, and (for some municipalities) minimum staff/resident ratios. As seen, nursing homes are not obliged to adhere to these guidelines, nor are the guidelines enforced in any strict form within (and, it would seem outside) our municipality. Though nursing homes must relate to these guiding principles, they maintain a degree of autonomy in deciding total number and composition of caring staff. As such, and despite a structural framework aimed at universality, variation between nursing homes *can* and *does* occur. Nursing homes in Norway vary in total number of caring staff; relative number of the respective professional groups (registered nurses, assisting nurses and assistants); total number of caring staff per resident; and total number of the respective professional groups per resident. Although nursing homes follow a similar overall pattern of distribution of staff on different shifts, there are also variations in this area, making, in effect, some nursing homes better staffed than others in total or, for instance, in the evening. The variation in staffing patterns between nursing homes is significant for staff and residents alike. Staffing patterns affect other mentioned factors, but are also affected by them. Staffing patterns relate to the size of nursing homes; larger nursing homes tend to be staffed differently, most notably by having less total number of caring staff per resident than smaller. Staffing patterns can be related to physical layout in the sense that having a sensible and functional physical environment might diminish the workload for caring staff, leading, potentially, to the need for less caring staff. Similarly, staffing patterns can be related to the level of sick leave in several ways. Low levels of staffing, in general or at specific times, might lead to increased levels of sick leave, while the experience of workload, the work environment in general and the practices of nursing homes towards filling vacancies, might influence the caring staff's threshold for short-term sickness absence. Staffing patterns can also be connected to treatment options and facilities in nursing homes. The offer of specialized treatment regimens, intravenous treatment or laboratory testing, for instance, implies specialized staff at hand, and could influence the composition of staff in nursing homes offering such treatments. In short, staffing patterns are influenced by and influence other mentioned factors, in involved and potentially different ways. Staffing patterns also affect the working conditions of staff and the everyday lives of residents. As will be discussed, staffing levels are highly significant for the practices of caring staff, in general and for specific occurrences such as acute illness of residents. However, the staffing level by itself, can be seen as a «surrogate marker» for decisions of hospitalization, while other factors, most notably *experience of staff*, can have a more direct influence.

Coverage of physicians has, according to the reviewed literature, produced varying effects for rates of hospitalizations. There seems, however, to be agreement on the general point that inaccessibility of physicians is influential for practices of hospitalizations (Jablonski et. al. 2007, McCloskey et al. 2011); if physicians are not present, in the evening for instance, hospitalizations tend to increase. Types of employment for physicians can be seen as a direct consequence of the structural framework to which nursing homes must relate, as presented earlier. Municipalities provide physicians' services to nursing homes who do not employ physicians directly, and provide physicians' services in addition to the hours covered by the nursing home physicians. However, this structural framework does not strictly bind nursing homes. National regulations do not stipulate *how* physicians should be employed, minimum physician hours per resident (besides an unsanctioned recommendation of being «responsible»), or *when* and *how* physicians should be available during and outside their allotted time in nursing homes. Municipalities can, meanwhile, provide norms for recommended coverage (for public institutions), and provide physicians' services for public (and willing) private institutions, such as in our municipality. Still, they do not determine (or impose sanctions on) *how* physicians are employed by private institutions (if not through the municipal agreement), or *when and how* physicians should be available outside time spent at the nursing home (while determining when they are available *at* the nursing homes for public and some private institutions). Nor does our municipality impose sanctions on deviations from their norm, or otherwise strictly enforce the norm. Consequently, private nursing homes can employ physicians independently, private homes can offer physicians more hours per resident than the municipality can provide, and (all – both private and public) have different arrangements about how and when to communicate with him/her when not available at the nursing home. As such, variation *can* and, as we shall see, *does* occur.

Treatment options, covering nursing homes´ offering of medical or other health-related treatment regimens, vary considerably between nursing homes. Such treatment regimens can include intravenous therapy, x-rays and laboratory blood tests taken «in house». As a general point, variation in nursing homes' access to and use of «services» has been addressed in research relating to its influence on decisions on hospitalizations (Bottrell et al. 2001, Kayser-Jones et al. 1989, Laging et al. 2015, Lamb et al. 2011), including both in-house and external treatment options. It is argued that nursing homes vary considerably regarding both *«available technologies»* and *«personnel resources»* allocated to resources (Bottrell et al. 2001). Cross-jurisdictional comparisons on this area are problematic, however, as the organization of treatment options varies considerably. Our nursing homes vary in what treatment options, if any, the homes offer, and in how they generally relate to the topic of extensive and/or advanced medical treatment of their residents. While only three nursing homes within the sample offer intravenous therapy, all nursing homes have some sort of arrangement for laboratory tests, either taken in-house, through a physician´s office or through a local hospital (implying, for the latter two cases, a longer procedure than for the former). Our nursing homes also related very differently, if at all, to the requisitions of external x-ray services: some planning for x-ray services to be performed in-house, some opting to transport residents for x-rays. In general, our nursing homes vary regarding having a strategy or policy towards treatment options, and how explicit such a strategy or policy is communicated to and among the caring staff.

The positioning of nursing homes towards treatment options should, in my opinion, be viewed as individual, unique and as non-determined by their respective characteristics. However, some connections between treatment options and other institutional conditions can still be found. The offer of treatment options relates to the size of nursing homes; the larger tend to have more treatment alternatives than the smaller, particularly intravenous therapy, perhaps as a result of economy of scale. Treatment options *can* also, in a far subtler way, be connected to ownership; private institutions may have lesser bureaucratic hurdles with regard to the requisitioning/purchasing of equipment needed, and may also have developed a culture of seeking new knowledge not always present in many public institutions. However, a related area seems to have a more direct effect on treatment options: the relative financial well-being of the respective institutions. Nursing homes need funds, in addition to initiative, to be able to acquire and maintain treatment options. Lastly, as already made clear, treatment options can influence staffing patterns; having a high level of treatment options necessitates a skilled group of caring staff. The prevalence of treatment options can also make a nursing home more attractive to skilled applicants, and can also lead to further training of current staff. At the same time, treatment options can *be influenced* by staffing patterns; caring staff with a high level of formal education tend to seek out alternative treatment regimens, as illustrated at several nursing homes within our sample. Especially at two of our nursing homes, Acre Woods and Emerald Gardens, registered nurses and assisting nurses would lobby the institutional or unit leadership for the introduction of a new treatment regimen.

The factors discussed in this chapter will be revisited throughout the analysis, adding detail and nuances, while a more theoretical discussion of *how practice affects and is affected* will be given in Chapter 9. Two initial outcomes can be outlined already at this point, paving the way for the succeeding analysis.

Generally, the influences on practices in nursing homes are complex: they influence differently, at different times and different places; their effects are non-determinant. Consequently, the study of what practices, such as hospitalizations, are affected by, should include analyses of a multitude of potentially relevant factors, including their relational, and not simply respective, influence. Based on such an understanding a preliminary model of the relationship between the structural framework, (a multitude of) institutional conditions and practices can be drafted:

This preliminary, generic model outlines the general dynamics of influence for nursing homes, rather than depicting a static and/or precise mode of influence for specific nursing homes. It points to tendencies rather than rules. I will, however, argue that the tendencies outlined are relevant for all nursing homes, both regarding the relationship between a structural framework, institutional

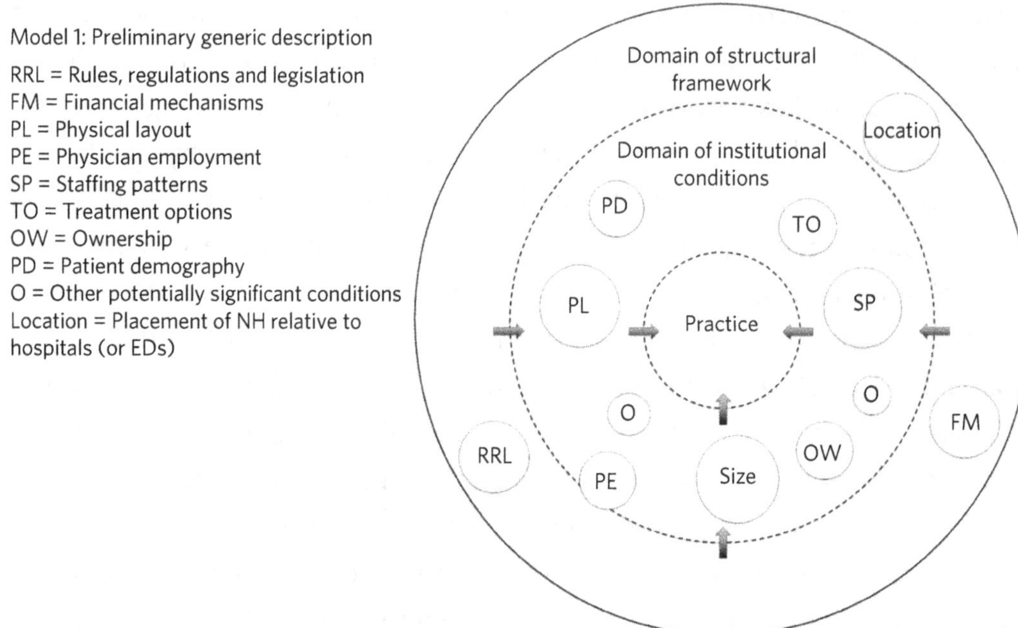

conditions and practice, the institutional conditions which are at play and the given emphasis on relevance of the respective institutional conditions (as illustrated through size of circles).

The structural framework and institutional conditions discussed, which I will argue are the most promising given the sample and its context, do not, collectively and respectively, determine practices such as hospitalization. Rather they provide premises from which practice is generated.

5.3. Meeting a resident: the hospitalization of Rita

Rita

Rita, a resident of Acre Woods, was, as Alice, (see Chapter 10.4), a resident who did not take up much space and did not make much fuss. She was small in size and seldom craved attention either from residents or staff. She did not seem to be cognitively impaired, perhaps except being somewhat absentminded, and had all her senses intact; she was keenly aware of what happened around her, although without showing much interest. Her physical state was another matter; she was frail (without, to my knowledge, suffering from a specific diagnosis), weak, for lack of a better word. When walking, she would take small steps shuffling her feet quietly one before the other, almost as if being careful not to disturb those around her. The caring staff would often pay attention to where and how Rita was seated, helping her rise, always with the possibility of Rita falling in the back of their minds.

When talked to, Rita would give clear and comprehensible answers, but she never started a conversation and did not seek attention. To the surprise of a caring staff member who did not know her, she would give clear, matter-of-fact answers when spoken to, sometimes also correcting the staff member's ways of doing things. She came into the large common room for meals, but stayed in her room at most other times. Sometimes she would sit in a chair in the corner of the main common room, alone, keeping her thoughts to herself. In my eyes, she seemed content, perhaps at ease with there not being much more to her existence, waiting for the inevitable end.

During a morning report meeting in *the unit*, all attention was directed towards Rita, who had fallen the previous evening. According to the assisting unit leader, Rita had suffered a fracture in her femur and needed an operation. An assistant had heard Rita cry out the previous evening, and had entered her room, finding her in pain. An ambulance had been called immediately and they had taken her to the local hospital.

Two days later, the assisting unit leader updated the caring staff about Rita's situation. She had been operated on, apparently successfully, but had had to stay at the hospital a little while longer for observation. Rita had caught pneumonia, which, combined with the operation, was a cause for great concern. Whether or not Rita had caught pneumonia before or after her fall was uncertain. The assisting unit leader added, this time opening the floor for feedback and discussion as opposed to simply informing the rest, that Rita´s fall might have been caused by her catching pneumonia, making her even more physically frail than before. She asked the others how they had found Rita´s state in the days leading up to the fall. An assisting nurse said that she was in poor condition, but did not know about her having pneumonia. Another said that the pneumonia might have been in the beginning stages, and had intensified since arriving at the hospital.

A week later, Rita returned to the unit. She was now temporarily bound to a wheelchair, and mostly stayed in her room. She seemed to have recovered somewhat from the pneumonia, as she dined with the rest of the residents in the main common room on several occasions. Her state quickly deteriorated though. At the evening report meeting about a week after her return, a registered nurse, who had discussed the matter with the physician and the unit leader, informed the others that the end was approaching for Rita. Two of the assisting nurses nodded, giving the impression that they knew about Rita's state. It seemed that Rita had once again caught pneumonia, and that treatment did not help. She was permanently bedridden, and *has stopped taking nourishment*[2], according to the registered nurse. One of the more experienced assisting nurses nodded, as if concurring, and added: *She has given up now*. The report meeting ended in a somber mood, as the caring staff seemed to accept that there was nothing to be done for Rita, aside from providing comfort.

Two days later, Rita´s closest family members, who had already been informed of the situation and had been to visit Rita, were called upon to be with Rita for her last hours. An extra assisting nurse was called on duty for the night-shift, to help provide Rita with palliative care. In addition, the night duty registered nurse was available in the unit for most of the night. Rita died, as she had lived in the unit, quietly, the same night.

---

2   Translated from the Norwegian «Stoppet å ta til seg næring». «Nourishment» refers to the intake of both food and liquids.

The ambiguity of «hospitalizations»

Hospitalizations, I will argue, are seldom easily identified or measurable events, clearly separated from other events, or even the normalcy of nursing home life. «Hospitalization» is not necessarily easily measurable for the researcher, nor is it easily identifiable and resolved by the practitioner.

Hospitalizations are difficult to concretize because of potentially different interpretations of what is defined as acute, of the places to which nursing home transfers are made (hospitals and/or emergency wards) and of the degree of treatment and time of stay at the receiving institution. *Measuring* hospitalizations, for the researcher, can therefore be problematic, as both interpretations of what a hospitalization is and the structural conditions to which nursing homes must relate, may differ. Measuring rates of hospitalizations for the sake of measurement can become a fool's errand; an undertaking of measuring that which might not be measurable and comparing that which is not comparable (or not comparable to others' comparison).

Even though hospitalizations can take different shapes, *understanding the dynamics behind (potential) hospitalizations* is a relevant undertaking, as different understandings can be useful as a starting point for understanding *variation* in practices, in addition to different forms of the empirical phenomenon itself. As many decisions on whether to hospitalize or not are filled with ambivalence, implying a multitude of different skills on the part of those involved, the researcher studying hospitalizations should include potential rather than actual hospitalizations.

6.1. What is a hospitalization?

As mentioned in Chapter 4, a definition of «hospitalization from nursing homes» is often missing in the research literature. The missing definition is problematic, especially because most of the cited studies compare findings with other studies. Potentially, hospitalization *can* be understood in different ways. When analyzing the research literature, it also becomes apparent that hospitalization *is* treated differently. To simplify: it is often unclear if studies on hospitalization are addressing the same understanding of the phenomenon. Potential differences of inclusion and exclusion are often not discussed.

6.1.1. Acute and non-acute hospitalizations

First, hospitalizations from nursing homes can be considered acute, or not. Acute hospitalizations are generally considered to be hospitalizations where residents of nursing homes suddenly (but not necessarily unexpectedly) become ill, and where the severity of the illness is considered to be such that treatment at the hospital rather than in the nursing home is warranted. Separating acute and non-acute hospitalizations seems, at first glance, to be useful as they clearly pose considerably different procedures and dilemmas for staff, and entail greatly different consequences for residents. Many residents of nursing homes need to visit the hospital, regularly and irregularly, for planned controls, checkups and evaluations. This can be connected to a more or less chronic diagnosis, cancer for instance, or to a less serious and passing diagnosis not considered acute, but still serious enough to warrant a visit to the hospital. The extent to which nursing homes use hospitals for such services can vary based on what the nursing home can offer in medical treatment, which again can be related to distance to hospitals. For some forms of treatment, however, nursing homes always have to refer to hospitals for planned controls and evaluations. Some residents visit hospitals for controls and checkups regularly for chronic diagnosis, perhaps once a month.

Scheduled controls and check-ups are common in nursing homes. Keeping in mind the age, frailty and comorbidity of most nursing home residents, many of them need medical treatment surpassing the expertise of the respective nursing homes. In many cases, this expertise is connected to chronic or recurrent diseases, making treatment at hospitals a continuous event. For the staff, such «hospitalizations» pose significantly different challenges than more acute cases. The main task is not to identify, understand and decide upon the nature of residents' ailments, and consequently whether or not the residents will benefit from the hospitalization, but is rather connected to organization and logistics, aspects that are not welcome challenges in the hectic schedule of nursing home life.

It should also be noted that if such controls and check-ups were defined as «hospitalizations», it would significantly change the rate of hospitalizations for many nursing homes. When including controls and check-ups (which were excluded from the original sample), one resident in a small nursing home suffering from a chronic diagnosis implying regular controls at the hospital, can result in a relatively high rate of hospitalizations for the entire nursing home, even when excluding all other hospitalizations.

However, not all hospitalizations can be neatly categorized as either «acute» or «non-acute». Many residents of nursing homes are in a more or less constant state of illness. The threshold of when their state of illness changes from what can be considered manageable to acute can therefore be gradual and diffuse. There may not be a defined, fixed period of time when this occurs, nor does it manifest itself as a specific episode. Thus, categorizing as «acute» or «non-acute» is difficult for the researcher and might even be misleading; caring staff might understand and define hospitalizations differently than the researcher, for instance. To complicate matters, caring staff might also have different understandings of both the severity and suddenness of residents' illnesses, often based on differences in experience and knowledge of specific residents. The diffuse and unclear development of residents' illnesses, then, also makes the understanding, evaluation and decisions about residents' well-being complicated and diffuse. Many residents are in a more or less constant state of being eligible for hospitalization, making the decision process for the staff ambiguous, constant and difficult:

Acre Woods, Monday morning, in the office of the unit leader. The unit leader updated me on the current events of the unit, after the weekend. She told me that a resident had died during the weekend, on late Friday evening. It was Ester, who *had just been with us a couple of months. It went fast,* she continued, *We had not noticed anything during the morning and early day. She had had a severe stroke already, from before, so it is not so easy to speak with her. She was already very marked by the stroke. Usually she just sat quietly, and didn't give much to us.* The unit leader continued her narrative of the events of the evening: since it was late evening, no registered nurses remained in the unit. When an assisting nurse had found Ester in her room, and suspected that something serious was wrong, she called the on-duty nurse. The on-duty nurse concluded that she was in a very bad state, perhaps even dying. She then called the family of Ester as quickly as possible, to ask them to come to see Ester, but it was too late. Ester died shortly thereafter. The on-duty nurse told the unit leader that they had talked about how to treat Ester, and was told that the family wanted as little treatment as possible, and that such a wish was in accordance with Ester's wishes as well. Still, not all was well, the unit leader told me. *She actually called me pretty soon after and was not satisfied. She was adamant about the fact that we should have noticed her earlier. I explained that it wasn't as easy as that. I don't know how we could have noticed it earlier.*

Another example can further illustrate the difficulties in interpreting residents and their ailments, even for experienced nursing home staff:

Acre Woods, Monday morning. I had been away from the unit the previous week, and knocked on the door of the unit leader, hopeful of getting an update of recent events. She greeted me, said that now was a good time and asked me to sit down. There had been one incident in particular the last week, she said. One of the oldest residents, Helga, had been hospitalized. On Monday morning, she had complained about her foot to an assisting nurse, when given morning care. The assisting nurse had not given it much thought as there was no visible damage to the foot. Some hours later, the unit leader continued, she complained again, when being served dinner. A registered nurse had taken a look and noticed that the foot had turned white. Immediately she suspected a thrombosis, I was told, in the area around the groin. A physician, not *ours*, she said, was called, looked at the resident and shared the concern of the registered nurse. *For cases such as this, there is just not that much we can do. It is difficult to see, if you know what I mean*, the unit leader explained, almost as a side note to her narrative. As a consequence, the resident had been sent directly to the nearest hospital. The unit leader concluded with another digression: *It was actually very similar to what has happened to Carina, twice actually, just in recent times. Perhaps we have become too sensitive towards this subject. I don't know.*

6.1.2. Hospitalizations to hospitals and emergency wards

The term hospitalizations *can* be applied to the referral of residents to not only hospitals, but also to emergency wards and/or departments. The latter may or may not be located in hospitals. Residents sent to an emergency ward and evaluated there may be further referred to a hospital (60 percent are, according to one source (Arendts & Howard 2010)), the likelihood of which is related to the location of a hospital in relation to the emergency ward, or they may be returned to the nursing home. Added to this, the function of emergency wards or departments can vary between or within jurisdictions, especially with regards to the level of treatment offered on-site. This variation might again be connected to the distance between emergency wards and hospitals, but also to differing jurisdictional policies and definition of «emergency wards». In our municipality, emergency wards are organized as autonomous entities, separated from hospitals. In other settings, however, defining whether or not a resident is transported to a hospital or an emergency ward might be problematic, especially when emergency wards are located in hospitals. Deciding whether or not the transfer of a resident to an emergency ward *should* be considered a hospitalization is probably even more problematic. This question relates not only to the operationalization, but also to the level of treatment received at emergency wards. Should a nursing home resident be considered hospitalized when she is sent from the nursing home to an emergency ward, or only when sent to a hospital? Or should the definition of «hospitalization» be more closely connected to level of treatment, rather than the name of the treatment facility? If so, how much treatment? What if the resident is returned to the nursing home after an examination either at the hospital or emergency ward? To paraphrase: if all transfers to emergency wards are excluded from our definition of hospitalization, a resident transferred to the emergency ward and receiving extensive treatment will not be considered a hospitalization, while a resident transferred to the hospital, and returned shortly after, might be considered a hospitalization, depending on whether or not time spent at the hospital is accounted for.

Acre Woods, Monday morning, report meeting. The meeting revolved around an incident happening the previous Friday. Many of the caring staff attending the morning report meeting had not been on shift since the incident, and therefore needed to be briefed. The oldest resident of the unit, Inga, had fallen at approximately 17.00, one of the registered nurses informed the rest. The registered nurse had been on shift when the incident occurred. According to the registered nurse, Inga, who can walk with assistance, had slid out of her chair, while in her room. Being alone when it happened, it took some time before anyone noticed, the registered nurse continued. She explained that they were not sure about what had happened and how serious it was, so they had called the emergency ward. Inga was transported to the emergency ward by ambulance, and had x-rays taken there. The x-rays came back negative, so she was returned to the nursing home, the registered nurse concluded. There was a brief silence, indicating that no one had any questions either about the incident or how to care for Inga after the fall.

6.1.3. Evaluation and treatment

Relating to the issue of emergency wards versus hospitals, hospitalization may refer to *the act* of resident transportation from nursing home to hospital (alternatively emergency ward), with no regard for the scope and/or content of the evaluation and treatment of the residents. Alternatively, hospitalization may refer to residents being *treated* at the hospital (alternatively emergency wards), thus excluding, for instance, residents being transported to the hospital, evaluated and sent back to the nursing home.

> Emerald Gardens, discussion with unit leader in her office. The unit leader: *We are starting to feel the effects of the Coordination Reform. Some residents are being sent back and forth. I guess that it has always been like this, but I feel that it is increasing. The most noticeable thing is that they return faster. One day and then back again. It's probably always been like this, but I think it has increased lately, especially when we send residents late in the evening or at night. Another thing I've noticed is the improper paperwork. It seems that when they return residents faster, they don't do the proper paperwork. Residents are sent back without a good overview of what has been done and what needs to be done.* After some further discussion about more recent changes, the unit leader brings up a specific resident: *You know about Asgeir. His disease means that he needs to go to the hospital a lot both for controls and treatment. It's very complicated. Especially now, because he's getting old and frail, there are other problems as well, that his disease has led to. Therefore he is constantly being sent back and forth, often too early, in my opinion.* I ask her what she thinks can or should be done about this. *I really don't know. You see, a big problem is the different doctors. Every time, there is a new doctor, so we have to start over again. It's extremely frustrating.*

The unit leader's comments relate to several aspects of hospitalizations, some already covered. How a nursing home relates to hospitalizations is not simply dependent on the respective characteristics of nursing homes and hospitals, but is also connected to local and national structural frameworks, such as locality of hospitals and, in this case, the Coordination Reform. The effect of the latter, the untimely return of residents to the nursing home, poses significant challenges for the staff of the nursing home, accentuated by the frailty of nursing home residents. The case of Asgeir also speaks to a point made earlier: residents transferred regularly to the hospitals for check-ups could significantly increase the rate of hospitalizations for the nursing home.

Should these latter examples be defined as hospitalizations? Most would agree that the example of Inga does not constitute a hospitalization; she was simply checked at the emergency ward, and returned to the nursing home immediately. But where should the line be drawn? An hour at the hospital, five hours, or twenty-four hours? Or, should the distinction between hospitalization and non-hospitalization rather be based on a division of evaluation and treatment, excluding residents being evaluated and including residents being treated for ailment or illness? This poses another question: what is «treatment»? Again, where should the line be drawn? The case of Asgeir illustrates the difficulty of isolating specific criteria: some of his transfers could be construed as check-ups, while others implied a more comprehensive treatment regimen. The example also highlights another point, not discussed previously: if the resident is returned to the hospital immediately after being sent to the nursing home, should it be considered two separate hospitalizations or one continuous event? As for the topics of acute versus non-acute and hospitals versus emergency wards, the majority of the research literature does not concern itself explicitly with these latter questions. Hospitalization is usually understood as a resident being transported from the nursing home to a hospital, with sporadic emphasis on time of stay at hospitals (or emergency wards) and even less emphasis on the degree of treatment during the stay at the hospital (or emergency ward).

Cloud House, 11.15 on a weekday. I am in the office of the unit leader who previously has told me that she *has some information for me.* I sit down opposite her, while she sits behind her desk with the computer monitor on. She tells me that they had an *incident* earlier, for which she was not present. She has, however, been briefed about it, she says while indicating that the information is also available on the electronic journal on her computer. While giving an account of the incident, she reads from the journal, and does not sway from the detailed and «objective» accounts of the incident: *She had a fall and also had a cut under the eye and a swelling as a result of that. Did not complain about pain. The emergency ward was contacted for consultation. Suspicion of hip fracture.* When finished reading from the journal, she adds some background information for my benefit: *Sometimes the registered nurses can handle the situation, especially with wounds and similar things, so they don´t have to contact the emergency ward. But in this case, it was the uncertainty of the hip fracture that led to the decision to call the emergency ward. Sometimes the emergency ward can help a lot by phone. But we can also do a lot here. So what happened in the end was that the resident was sent to the emergency ward, based on the advice of the people they talked to. Later she was returned here by ambulance without going to the hospital. They concluded that she was very sore but did not have a fracture.*

When considering the totality of these challenges, defining and understanding hospitalization for the researcher becomes a complicated task. These challenges point not only to difficulties for the researcher, but also to the multifaceted and varied nature of hospitalization itself. Hospitalization is not a specific occurrence, easily categorized and generalized, but unfolds differently, has different scopes, different meaning definitions and severely different consequences for residents. That is, of course, not to say that some specific episodes fit well with the general notion of what a hospitalization is:

Acre Woods, evening-shift on a weekday. I have made an appointment with the on-duty registered nurse to follow her from 16.00 to 22.00[1]. I have not met the registered nurse before, but am familiar with the nursing home and the respective units. The following excerpts are from different, shorter periods during the shift, but all relate to the same episode.

17: We are in the office of the on-duty nurse, where we have talked about my project, the function of the on-duty nurse, and how a shift usually unfolds, for about thirty minutes. Meanwhile, she has been reading reports and notes from previous shifts. The phone rings. After a short conversation she tells me that one of the residents is ill. She would like to attend to the resident as soon as possible. The physician had seen to the resident earlier, sometime before 15.00, she tells me, and told the unit staff to wait until the next day. The registered nurse presents the information factually and soberly.

17.10: Together we go to the unit and greet an assisting nurse quickly (there are no registered nurses on shift in the unit). The on-duty nurse is led to the room of the resident. She enters while I remain at the entrance of the door. The on-duty nurse sees to the resident and tries to establish contact with her. The resident lets out some

---

1   All evening and night-shifts have one registered nurse serving as the duty nurse for the entire nursing home. The on-duty nurse is available for all units. Even though some of the units might have a registered nurse on staff for a given evening-shift, there will still be an on-duty nurse available. The registered nurses serving as on-duty nurses for evening and night-shift, do this exclusively. The duties of the on-duty nurse are many and varied. Their primary functions are to assist the units in acute instances, assist with the medication for units without proper formally educated staff on shift, to make rounds at all wards and to be responsible for fire safety.

guttural noises, but I am not sure if they are responses to the nurse or not. After about three minutes of evaluation from the nurse, where she continuously has eye or physical contact with the resident, the on-duty nurse asks the assisting nurse to fetch equipment to measure the resident's fever. The assisting nurse returns two minutes later and says that she cannot find the equipment. While the assisting nurse is present, the on-duty nurse rolls her eyes and shakes her head. She tells the assisting nurse to go to another unit to find what she needs. The assisting nurse returns three minutes later. Together they measure the resident's fever. The on-duty nurse says that it is 40 degrees, higher than what she would have liked. Meanwhile, the on-duty nurse attempts to establish contact with the resident, speaking to her while getting slurred responses, difficult to interpret. The on-duty nurse says that she believes that the resident has pains in her abdomen. She asks the resident several times about this. The on-duty nurse then asks the assisting nurse if the resident is usually this unresponsive, whereupon the assisting nurse says that she usually can express herself easily. This concerns the on-duty nurse, who decides to measure the EKG of the resident. We leave for the medicine room and collect the relevant apparatus. After measuring the EKG level of the resident, the on-duty nurse tells me that it is high, much higher than what she would have liked. She pauses for a couple of seconds, considering the situation, visibly concerned. At this point, the on-duty nurse seems to acknowledge a seriousness in the situation, not evident earlier. She noticeably increases her pace and chooses to focus solely on the resident, and not me or the assisting nurse. The on-duty nurse decides to give the resident Paracetamol rectally, and gets help from the assisting nurse. I leave the doorway and wait in the hallway until they return.

17.20: The on-duty nurse and I return to the office, where she intends to call the next of kin. She does not tell me a lot of what is going on, but rather gives short, descriptive explanations of her plans. After finding the information about the next of kin, the on-duty nurse talks to her for about five minutes. Again, in a factual manner she tells the next of kin what has happened to the resident, and says that she thinks it would be wise to call the on-duty physician at the emergency unit and ask for an immediate hospitalization, *directly to the hospital rather than the emergency unit*. When they have ended the conversation, she tells me that the next of kin agreed. As I interpret the conversation, the on-duty nurse advised an action and left the decision to the next of kin, while still emphasizing her point of view, so as to influence the decision of the next of kin. The on-duty nurse confirms this as she later expressed satisfaction with the fact that the next of kin agreed with her.

17.30: The on-duty nurse tries to call the on-duty physician at the emergency unit, but is told that the physician *has not reported for duty yet*. After considering the situation for a short while, she finds another phone number, which she tells me is the direct number for non-acute ambulances. She explains the situation over the phone to them. Her tone of voice has noticeably changed from talking to the next of kin; much more assertive and authoritative now. Without leaving the topic up for debate, she tells them that the resident needs to be hospitalized directly and immediately. It appears that they are debating whether or not the resident should be transported to the emergency unit first, rather than directly to the hospital. The on-duty nurse says that going to the emergency unit would be ineffective and unnecessary, as the situation for the resident warrants treatment at the hospital. She also says that going directly to the hospital is in the interest of the next of kin, and not just her. They continue debating this back and forth for a couple of minutes, while the on-duty nurse repeats her arguments, even more strongly towards the end. She ends the conversation. The on-duty nurse tells me that the ambulance is on the way. *Straight to the hospital?* I ask. *I hope so, but I´m not sure. I think I will get my way in the end*, she replies. She proceeds to write down information about the resident in her journal.

18.00: We return to the resident's room. The on-duty nurse measures her fever again. It remains high, approximately 45 minutes after getting medication, which unsettles the on-duty nurse.

18.10: Back at the office, the on-duty nurse once again phones the next of kin to given an update on the situation. Soberly, she runs through the turn of events, and adds that she thinks the resident will be sent to the hospital. She finishes the conversation by promising to phone again when she knows more.

18.25: The ambulance arrives. The on-duty nurse receives a phone call upon arrival and meets the two ambulance workers shortly thereafter by the elevator. They have brought a large stretcher. The ambulance workers and the on-duty nurse immediately go towards the resident's room, where the assisting nurse awaits them. The on-duty nurse and one of the ambulance workers discuss whether the resident should go to the hospital or the emergency ward. The ambulance worker, a young man, says that the on-duty nurse should call the nursing home physician, and that this is the correct procedure if they should go directly to the hospital. This visibly annoys the on-duty nurse. She raises her voice when she replies *He cannot come here now. And anyways,*

he can´t do the paperwork for a hospitalization from home. It´s just not very smart.
While this discussion is going on, the other ambulance worker has seen to the resident. After the conversation, the two gather and discuss between themselves, outside of hearing range from the rest of the people in the room. Shortly afterwards, they go over to the on-duty nurse, and discuss the matter with her, of which I can only hear parts. They then proceed to load the resident onto the stretcher, with the help of the assisting nurse. The resident lets out a small moan, but is otherwise unresponsive. She has not communicated with the ambulance workers since they arrived. While they leave, the on-duty nurse looks at me, smiles and says: *Well, that went well.*

18.50: We follow the ambulance workers to the elevator and return to the office. She calls the next of kin and updates her about the situation. Afterwards, she tells me that it is time for her rounds, which she was supposed to do earlier, but has not had time for because of the incident with the resident. I join her.

21.30: The on-duty nurse finally finds time for a small break. I join her in the canteen. After a while, she changes the topic of our conversation to the previous incident: *I didn´t like that they were so difficult.* I ask her what she means by that. *There really wasn´t any point in going back and forth so many times. They could have just listened to me from the beginning.* There is a small pause before she continues: *I don´t get why they insist on talking to the physician before deciding on a hospitalization. But, whatever, I got my way in the end, anyway.* After another short pause she continues by saying that she could have called the nursing home physician. *But there really wasn´t any point. She would have been hospitalized anyway, so it would just prolong the situation.* Another short pause. *You probably have noticed this already, but we usually get our way in the end! We always find a way, a lot of times a smart one, like getting it done without saying it straight out, you know.* She smiles while saying this, and ends her statement with a laugh.

In this case, the resident experienced an acute and severe physical crisis, for which she could not receive adequate treatment at the nursing home. She was transported to the hospital where she received extensive treatment, before dying two days later. As such, this particular instance serves as an example of «a typical hospitalization», consistent with the criteria discussed. This instance, both for the untrained observer and for the registered nurse, seemed like a clear-cut example where hospitalization was the only sensible outcome. Such is not always the case, however. Most decisions on whether to hospitalize or not, are difficult and filled with ambivalence, implying not only a multitude of different skills for those involved in the decisions, but also a change in approach for the researcher studying variation of practices connected to hospitalizations.

6.1.4. *Potential* hospitalizations

Hospitalizations appear seldom as precise and concrete. *Relating to* hospitalizations for caring staff, therefore, is not precise and concrete. Such an uncertainty, it will be argued, is emphasized by the lack of specific protocols and guidelines, resulting in uncertainty based on the consequent professional discretion (see Chapter 9). Adding to this, differences in structural and institutional conditions, such as size, vicinity of hospitals and continuity of physicians, can also influence both the occurrence and understanding of hospitalization. *Measuring* hospitalizations, in an attempt to analyze variation of hospitalizations between nursing homes, can therefore be problematic, as the local understanding of what a hospitalization is as well as the structural conditions influencing decisions of hospitalization, may differ.

I will argue that the researcher can transcend some of the challenges connected both to the measurement and to the analysis of variations by altering the general approach to the study of hospitalization commonly adopted. Instead of focusing on *actual* hospitalizations retrospectively, in an attempt to explain why these hospitalizations took place and why they differ from other hospitalizations, the researcher can benefit from focusing on the complicated and multi-faceted process of *decisions of hospitalization*, as represented by a minority of research. The suggested differences in approach are not just a matter of *when* potential hospitalizations should be studied, as prospective rather than retrospective, but also about empirical attention: all *potential* hospitalizations are relevant, not just *actual* hospitalizations. Given that practices, and consequently rates, of hospitalization differ between institutions, a resident that is hospitalized from one institution, might not, potentially, have been hospitalized from another. Not to include incidents when residents are considered for hospitalization but are not hospitalized is, in this sense, to leave out half of the picture:

> Acre Woods, morning on a weekday. Morning report meeting, which mainly revolved around a resident who had fallen ill the previous evening, has just ended. I remain

in the nurses' station, while a couple of assisting nurses finish their coffee before hurrying off to their designated tasks. Most of the caring staff have already left, some for the rooms of the residents, some for the large common room, and one for kitchen duty. The assisting unit leader, who led the morning report meeting in the unit leader's absence, enters after a short errand to talk to the physician. The assisting unit leader, a hardworking and diligent registered nurse, well-liked by staff, is at this point well known to me. Of all the staff in the unit, she has struck me as the most «professional» in the sense that she seldom presents opinionated statements, but rather sticks to a factual and somber presentation of events and explanations. She sits down beside me: *So, I thought you´d like to hear a little bit more about Mona.* She continues, still in a somber and factual manner: *Well, she had a pulmonary edema, suddenly from what we could tell. First, we gave her a diuretic through intravenous therapy.* I interrupt her, asking her about the technicalities of the procedure. She explains how the procedure is done with the objective of removing fluid from the lungs. *It helped,* she says, *but she didn´t get well, at least not immediately. That´s why the physician is here today, as well, to see her* (this was the day after the scheduled day of the physician at the unit). *I understand,* I reply. *Alternatively, we could have given her a diuretic through muscular injection, but we chose not to, as it takes longer to be effective,* she continues. I ask her if the family of the resident were involved. *Yes, we talked to them two times, actually, on the phone. The second time I talked to the son, who is a doctor. That is always a hassle.* She smiles after the last comment. After a short pause, signaling she had finished her account of the events, I ask her, *In regard to what we have talked about before, if treatment and decisions differ from place to place, do you think what you did would have been done at other places, given the same scenario?* She seems uncertain, at least I interpret her facial expression that way: *I don´t know. Others might have hospitalized, I guess, but I really don´t know. It´s always a possibility. We were satisfied, anyway, and were all in agreement.*

The suggested approach can account for the complicated and ambiguous dilemmas caring staff are influenced by when considering the well-being of their residents. Furthermore, an emphasis on *the process of the decisions of potential hospitalizations* is better suited than alternatives to account for the complicated relationship to structural frameworks and institutional conditions, discussed in the previous chapter and elaborated on later. Alas, such an approach will, as in our case, produce findings and connections that are themselves multi-faceted and complicated, as opposed to the determinant correlations produced in many of the retrospective analyses. I believe that such is the price of the study of the practices of hospitalizations, which *are* multi-faceted and complicated.

6.2. Meeting a resident: Whether or not to hospitalize Alexandra

Alexandra

Alexandra (see also excerpt in Chapter 8.2.) was one of the oldest residents at Acre Woods, relatively agile and mobile, walking around on her own, although with some difficulty. She did not, however, have much energy, often resting after a short walk, or indicating to the caring staff that she was tired and wanted to go to her room. She often seemed weary. Her mind, on the other hand, was ever-sharp, always paying close attention to her surroundings, always making a quick comment to the staff if they did not behave to her liking. Her weariness, meanwhile, seemed to affect her mood; she did not engage in long conversations with staff or residents, and chose to stay in her room most of the time. Like Rita (see Chapter 5.3.), Alexandra was physically weak and tired, and gave the impression, at least to me, of having lived long enough.

> After supper on a weekday, Alexandra had fallen in her room. An assistant had accompanied her from the large common room to her room for a nap (Alexandra often walked by herself with the aid of a walking frame, but sometimes got help from staff as well, especially when getting up from or into a chair or bed). The assistant had left Alexandra in a chair in her room while fetching a beverage from the kitchen area, when Alexandra, apparently, had risen by herself to lay down on her bed. The assistant found her by her bed shortly after, moaning and with a gash on her forehead. Alexandra was disoriented and could not account for what had happened or whether or not she was hurt elsewhere. After Alexandra was found, things transpired quickly. The assisting unit leader and another registered nurse arrived, and evaluated Alexandra's condition before calling the physician. From what I could understand at the time – not trying to interfere – the physician and the registered nurses had difficulty in ascertaining the gravity of Alexandra's condition: she could not talk, but seemed to be in pain, in addition to the cut on the forehead, which was bleeding profusely. Together they decided to call an ambulance to take Alexandra to the emergency unit for x-ray. The ambulance arrived shortly thereafter, taking Alexandra away.

The next day, the assisting unit leader, in the absence of the unit leader, updated me on the situation. *It was a good thing that we called (the ambulance), she suffered a fracture of the pelvic bone,* she explained. The assisting unit leader further explained that Alexandra had been brought back to the nursing home last night, as a pelvic fracture does not, at least in Alexandra's case, warrant an operation, as opposed to a femoral fracture. *So all, in all, a lucky thing!* she said, apparently relieved. She continued by explaining that the treatment regimen going forward would be rest and then gradual activation, to strengthen the area of the fracture: *But not yet, obviously, she is tired now, physically and mentally, no energy.* I asked whether they had considered not calling an ambulance at all. The assisting unit leader explained that they had considered not calling, but had decided that Alexandra needed to go to the emergency ward regardless, because of the cut on her forehead. The cut had been stitched, and was no longer a cause for concern.

Alexandra was discussed at the report meeting later that day and the days to come. The assisting unit leader, who usually expressed herself with confidence and professional certainty, was uncertain of how to proceed and wanted to discuss the matter with the rest of the caring staff members. The emergency ward had informed the nursing home that Alexandra needed *gradual activation and pain relief* to secure a swift and complete recuperation, but had not, according to the assisting unit leader, specified when and how the activation should start. The following discussion did not provide any definitive answers, as no one seemed to be certain when Alexandra would be ready to start the process of activation. They decided to discuss the matter of the amount and form of pain relief further with the unit physician, while the matter of activation had to be addressed later, as they had to see whether and when Alexandra felt better. It was clear that the matter of pain relief was, at least in part, within the physician's domain, while the matter of activation was not, being a matter within the domain of the caring staff.

One week later, Alexandra's state had not improved considerably. She was still weak, immobile and still suffering from the consequences of the fall, to the surprise of some of the caring staff. Others, at least two experienced assisting nurses, were not surprised, saying, in hindsight, that they *could have said that this would happen* and that *it is obvious that she had given up.* At a report meeting later in the week, Alexandra's case was addressed again, this time by the unit leader. She said that it appeared that the end was approaching for Alexandra, and that it was *important that everyone should come to terms with this, at this point.* It seemed that there was no hope left for the recovery of Alexandra, making the statement from the unit leader «the official» mark of a change in approach towards her. They discussed Alexandra's state together for about 10 minutes, agreeing with the unit leader's decision. An assisting nurse said that it was noticeable how Alexandra no longer had any interest in leaving her bed, *I don't think she sees the point anymore.* The assisting unit leader agreed, before pointing out that there was another disadvantage to Alexandra staying in bed: bedsores, to which everyone was asked to pay close attention. An assisting nurse changed the subject by asking how Alexandra's liking for red wine should be addressed when given pain relief. The assisting unit leader dismissed the potential issue, by saying that she could have as much wine as she wanted; *even though she is on strong sedatives, wine is still ok, in fact, it is probably better to offer her more wine and less sedatives.* The unit leader took the floor again, saying she had talked to a daughter of Alexandra, who had come to terms with the fact that the end was approaching for her mother. The daughter had agreed with the notion of no «excess treatment» for Alexandra, including no hospitalization when that time came.

I did not come back to the unit for another five days. When back and going down the hallway, I noticed that the door to Alexandra's room was open. A staff member from the nursing home's maintenance department was changing the linoleum on the floor, while all other furniture and signs of Alexandra were gone. Alexandra had died two days before and the nursing home was expecting a new resident the following day. A strong smell of glue had spread across the hallway, while all traces of Alexandra were gone.

Part two of the analysis: the premises of practice

While part one of the analysis has provided a preliminary analysis of the empirical phenomenon and treatment of hospitalization, part two will concern itself with more general aspects both of our nursing homes and the doxic idea, notion and representation of «the nursing home». The gaze will be raised from the specific analysis of hospitalizations to a broader empirical object, towards understandings of what the nursing home is and should be, based on several opposing tensions (Chapter 7), and representations of «the hardship and toil» of the nursing home (Chapter 8). Representations of staff and residents will be analyzed in relation to the characteristics of residents and staff at *our* nursing homes.

The analysis of the nursing home is divided in two parts. In part one we will move beyond «commonsensical» representations of the nursing home, through the construction of dichotomies serving as tensions in a complex and varied institution (Chapter 7). In part two representations made by its primary agents; caring staff members will be presented and analyzed (Chapter 8).

Simultaneously, we will move from abstract understandings of the nursing home (Chapter 7) to the inner workings of *our* nursing homes (Chapter 8).

Understandings of the nursing home and the resident, in combination with the forms of rules and regulations to which caring staff must relate, serve as premises from which practice is created and implemented. These elements provide a framework from which institutional autonomy can potentially thrive, allowing also for *variation of practice.*

Understanding the nursing home

What meaning and understanding is attributed to the notion of «the nursing home» by the respective agents and what does such a meaning and understanding entail for staff and residents?

The social fact or phenomenon of study must be constructed to avoid the illusion of immediate knowledge, readily available and alluring for the researcher. However, distancing oneself from the immediate knowledge is a daunting task: «*Everyday notions are so tenacious that all techniques of objectification have to be applied in order to achieve a break that is more often proclaimed than performed*» (Bourdieu et al. 1991: 13). This *break*, a main objective for Bourdieu's social scientist, can be understood to be a factor on different levels: the researcher should aim to achieve an *epistemological* break from prevalent and distorting scientific discourses and the doxa they represent, but also a break from «*ordinary language and certain scholarly uses of ordinary words* [which] *constitute the main vehicle for common representations of society*» (Ibid.: 14). The latter point also implies a methodological break; primarily from relying exclusively on native accounts as sources for understanding and explanations of social dynamics (Bourdieu 2012: 18-19, see also Chapter 1).

For our purposes, in studying the nursing home, *the break* implies distancing ourselves from the doxic notions and representations of the nursing home, as presented and acted upon both by scientific discourses, public and official accounts, and agents operating inside or at the boundaries of the actual institutions, as well as a methodological break from relying solely on natives' accounts of the nursing homes:

> «*If these epistemological preliminaries are ignored, there is a great risk of treating identical things differently and different things identically, of comparing the incomparable and failing to compare the comparable, because in sociology even the most objective*

«data» are obtained by applying grids (age groups, income brackets, etc.) which involve theoretical presuppositions and therefore overlook information which another construction of the facts might have grasped.» (Bourdieu et al. 1991: 36-37)

As such, by breaking from commonsensical understanding of the nursing home, by way of constructing the object «the nursing home» (Petersen 1996), we might be able to grasp a sociological understanding which surpasses that of an instrumental comparison of characteristics of nursing homes (which might also be an exercise in *«comparing the incomparable»*) as a means of explaining the result of a given practice. Such a break can leave us, I believe, capable of analyzing from where practice is created.

Two aspects of the nursing home will be highlighted as particularly dominating; that of the nursing home as being *the last home of residents* and *the nursing home as an institution*. I will argue that these aspects are thoroughly embedded in a doxic notion of the nursing home, since the overarching structural framework, or the objective conditions to which nursing homes relate (to use Bourdieu´s terminology), *allows it to be.* That being said, within the overarching doxic notion of the nursing home, a battle of sorts ensues: tension arises from being betwixt and between an institution and a home, and being between an ideology of medicine and treatment, and «care». Removed from a commonsensical understanding of the nursing home, then, we can construct dichotomies or tensions, to which nursing homes are invariably connected, conceptually *and* in everyday practice. Constructing dichotomies or tensions can be a productive analytical undertaking, in part because they are seldom presented as such (Armstrong 2013), thus emphasizing that which is contested within a given field (Bourdieu 2012). Such tensions, for our purposes, are not simply theoretical constructs, but also constitute a framework for agents operating within the nursing home; caring staff are constantly and continuously torn between opposing interests, values and ideologies.

7.1. Tales of «the nursing home»

The nursing home as an idea or a notion has many elements or aspects attributed to it. Some, I believe are of particular importance, both for representations of it (as grounded in a doxa) and experiences of it (as through the everyday life of staff and residents).

7.1.1. The nursing home as the last place of residency

Nursing homes are, primarily, where elderly go to live the remainder of their lives when other options are scarce or non-existing. Many residents, perhaps most, reside in nursing homes out of necessity, because there are no other options. Few have, on their own accord, chosen to live in nursing homes; for them the nursing home is the only alternative. From the perspective of the healthcare sector, as for many families of residents, the same also holds true: they see few, if any, realistic alternatives for the care of elderly people in need of physical and emotional support, besides nursing homes. Potential residents are cognitively or physically impaired, often both, to a degree where they cannot care for themselves or stay at home with assistance from visiting nurses. Families are seldom capable of caring properly for their elderly family members; they do not have the time or the medical competence to do so in a way deemed proper by themselves or society in general. The public discourse about nursing homes, in Norway and internationally, *has deeply incorporated this notion* of the absolute necessity of long-term institutional care for the elderly. The need for nursing homes and the idea that the nursing home is the only viable option for many residents is more or less taken for granted. Nursing homes are considered a necessity; a necessary by-product of the modern family structure and increased lifespan of the elderly. Both from the perspective of family members of potential nursing home residents and the general public discourse about eldercare, there are no viable options aside from nursing homes. This necessity, the accuracy of which will not be debated here, should not, however, keep us from being reminded that nursing homes can be a challenging, difficult, hard, confusing, alienating, lonely and painful experience for those who live there. Such an elementary understanding of nursing homes is often missing from the public and academic discourse about nursing homes. *The necessity of nursing homes* should therefore not be reduced to a societal necessity, but is first and foremost a necessity for its residents, which can be unwanted.

7.1.2. The nursing home as an institution

The nursing home is also *an institution*. Residents of nursing homes sleep, eat, play, and interact with insiders and outsiders, all in the confines of the institution, all trademarks of the «total institution» described by Goffman (1961: 11).

As will be discussed, the institution always has its sets of rules, routines and structures, to which residents and staff must adhere. The nursing home institution also has an involved relationship with the concept of medicalization, which is not as prevalent as in many other (total) institutions. From the perspective of the resident, meanwhile, the institution is total; their entire life revolves around it, and many must be terminally ill to escape it, but alas only to another institution, the hospital. For many nursing homes, primarily depending on size, the institution is comprised of several «mini-institutions», the units. For the resident, there is little physical or social mobility between the mini-institutions, while at least some of the staff have more mobility between units. The nursing home is also an institution from the perspective of families, staff and the governing bodies, albeit an institution they can frequent more or less as they please. The «totality» of the institution is relative, in other words: a total institution for its residents, a place of work for some, and a necessary public support institution for others.

As an institution the nursing home must relate to official rules, norms and expectations from the outside world. From the outside world, a nursing home has an official status, in the sense that it is publicly recognized and validated as a «nursing home», based on the fulfillment of certain characteristics. The nursing home needs to have the appearance, organizational characteristics and staff positions of a «nursing home» for it to be eligible to fill its societal function: the caretaking of the frail elderly. In other words, the nursing home is filled with content, from the eyes of the outsider; it is supposed to be a certain institution somewhere between the medicalized hospital and a home (Jacobsen 2004). In this sense, the outsider has an idea of what the nursing home is, even if they have never visited one. The outsider also has a clear understanding about the absolute necessity of nursing homes.

As an institution, the nursing home shares similar traits across jurisdictions, being regional and national. The specific definitions of the institution for long-term care for the elderly vary somewhat between countries, and there are varying definitions within countries, as we have seen for Norway. Nonetheless, many use the term «nursing home». The content of the term «nursing home» naturally also varies both within and between countries, especially in regard to organizational structure. Still, based on the extensive research literature on nursing homes in different jurisdictions and fieldwork at two nursing homes respectively in the United Kingdom, Canada and the United States, the general characteristics as well as the more subjectively experienced «spirit» of nursing homes are surprisingly similar. The similarities of nursing homes across jurisdictions are more striking than differences. The decisions, dilemmas and choices discussed in the following will therefore resonate outside a Norwegian and Scandinavian context.

However, I will still argue that the nursing home as an institution is particularly embedded as a collective perception in Norway: Norwegians have a distinct idea of what a nursing home is and should be, as well as the importance of the institution. Such a homology can be attributed to the high number of nursing homes, the relative homogeneity in ownership status of nursing homes compared to other countries as well as the general level of public governance in Norway. As such, the doxic notion of the nursing home is firmly established in a Norwegian context. The doxic notion of the nursing home *can be* firmly established, because of the particular contextual and structural framework surrounding it:

> «*In a determinate social formation, the stabler the objective structures and the more fully they reproduce themselves in the agents' dispositions, the greater the extent of the field of doxa, of that which is taken for granted. When, owing to the quasi-perfect fit between the objective structures and the internalized structures which results from the logic of simple reproduction, the established cosmological and political order is perceived not as arbitrary, i.e. as one possible order among others, but as self-evident and natural order which goes without saying and therefore goes unquestioned, the agents' aspirations have the same limits as the objective conditions of which they are the product.*»
> (Bourdieu 2012: 165-6)

The relative «*stable objective structure*» of the Norwegian healthcare sector in general, the development of nursing homes as the preferred form of long-term care for the elderly and the significant public involvement in the nursing home sector, allow for an «*extension of the field of doxa*», making the idea of «the nursing home» largely taken for granted. The relatively «*stable objective structure*» does not imply, however, that the field of opinion that it resides within is uncontested, or that actual practice at the nursing homes is determined by it.

7.2. Tensions of the nursing home

The nursing home as *a last home* and as *an institution* can be described as significant and, in part, taken-for-granted aspects of the nursing home.

Respectively meanwhile, they include elements that are problematized and contested. *The last home* and *the institution* have within them embedded elements that are opposing and contested, not necessarily visible at first glance. When deconstructed, *tensions* between opposing ideals, norms, ideologies and specific decisions can be found within the notion of the nursing home. These tensions can be found on a conceptual level *and*, most importantly for our purpose, in the everyday life of specific nursing homes. The primary tension is to be found between «the home» (in the sense of private and individualized, rather than a last home) and «the institution» (in the sense of a structured and governed bureaucracy, rather than a total institution). Behind this tension, other, related tensions can be found, most notably that between *professionalization* and *personal autonomy*, and between *medicalization* and «care».

7.2.1. The nursing home as an institution and a home

On one level, the nursing home is in a constant and complex flux between «*home*» and «*bureaucracy*» (Jacobsen 2005). The nursing home as «*a home*» can also be contrasted to «*the public*», as thoroughly documented elsewhere, resulting, for instance in opposing expectations of the use of common rooms (Hauge 2004). The home can also be given varied attributes and connotations, and, depending on one's perspective, be dichotomized differently; to «*the public*», «*the institutional*» or to «*the civic*», for instance (Ibid.). With the primary objective of understanding variations between nursing homes in mind, I propose to view the nursing home as *a home* as dichotomized by an external and internal need for and a tendency to bureaucratize the institution, in line with similar understanding from Slagsvold (1986) and Jacobsen (2005). The nursing home institution can be viewed as bureaucratized, for example in the sense of having procedures and an organizational format that are structured and (supposedly) followed. Such procedures and organization are seen as the result of (local and/or generic) managerial planning, aimed at securing efficiency (including cost-efficiency) and being beneficial for the organization, staff and residents. Consequently, procedures are reported on and outcomes are measured, to ensure that operations go according to plan. Such an emphasis stands opposed to, or at least in a competitive relationship with the idea of the nursing home as *a home*. The home is not cost-efficient, work is not measured and evaluated against output, nor are the activities in the home routinized as strictly as they are in the institution.

As such, nursing homes are simultaneously *a home* and *a bureaucratized institution*, with internal and external demands for structure and efficiency. Such a dichotomy can best be illustrated by variations in aesthetics (understood broadly), relating again to another dichotomy; the aesthetic of *the home* and *the hospital.*

In effect, nursing homes approach such a dichotomy in very different ways. The primary resistance to the various forms of bureaucratization in nursing homes comes from the widespread notion that *the home* is an ideal for nursing homes. Nursing homes are meant to have a feel, an atmosphere and the appearance of being somehow connected to a home, rather than an anonymous and clinical institution. Such sentiments, described as the «*aesthetics of being homelike*» (Lundgren 2000), can cover specific ways of decorating nursing homes as well as assumptions and concepts relating to a «good» home (Ibid.: 109-110). Martin (2002) presents a similar division, between «*homey*» and «*institutional facilities*». In accordance with my understanding, Martin treats aesthetics as more than decoration and physical objects, aesthetics is also connected to an ambiance, or the «*spirit of a place*»; «*...the corpus of sensory perceptions in and reactions to residential organizations for the elderly. This phrase refers to an organization's ambiance and emotional climate, including its members' and my sensate and emotional reactions to the physical and social context*» (Ibid. 863). Furthermore, «*the spirit of a place*» is not seen as random or as if appearing from a vacuum, rather it is seen as being produced both by «*unreflective practices*» and «*reflective praxis*» (Ibid.).

Returning to our setting, the sentiment of *homelike* as an ideal is shared by all those directly involved with nursing homes: residents, caring staff, administration and families. The home is always a part of the nursing home, and should be so; it *should* be something to strive for. While some attributes of the home, most notably «the spirit», are as difficult to create as they are perceptible to the visitor, other attributes, adornments and furniture for instance, are easier to manipulate. Variation in the appearance of nursing homes is no more apparent than in the decoration of common areas, primarily hallways and dining areas; the main areas for leisure time for residents and for staff-resident interaction. The styles of nursing home decoration range from that of mock antique shops (where every possible space is covered by objects of «old times», highlighted by warm colors (yellow, and pink), perfumed scents and music), to the polar extreme, the mock hospital (with long, sterile hallways with no unnecessary decoration, bright and neutral colors (white, grey), no music, and the smell of washing detergent). Somewhere between these extremes, we find our nursing homes, each one with its individual interpretation of «homelike», each one with its individual feel and atmosphere. Some nursing homes have an explicit policy in regard to decoration, expressing a desire for a home-like feel, or downplaying such in an attempt to be perceived as «a serious institution», while others do not, and let the aesthetic of the common area live its own life, depending on staff initiative.

How the administration and caring staff choose to present their nursing home's appearance, and keep in mind that the staff has omnipotent power over residents when it comes to this matter, speaks not only to how the nursing homes want to be perceived, but also to how they perceive *the nursing home*. The aesthetic of the nursing home, «*the spirit of a place*», is in this sense connected to how staff position their nursing homes, somewhere along a scale where the home and the institution, and the aesthetics of homelike and hospital-like are the extremes. The appearance of nursing homes is a comment on what nursing homes should be, and therefore a comment on how the values of *home* and *institution* are perceived. Nursing homes position themselves, implicitly and explicitly, every day, along this scale. It is important to note, however, that nursing homes do not appear as archetypes; they do not fit into one or the other extreme variant, they do not incorporate fully the value of one extreme and neglect the other. Nursing homes are always betwixt and between a home and a bureaucratized institution. They always borrow elements from the home and the institution *simultaneously*, leading, as we shall see, to practices that are always between the influence of the need for «personal attention» and «professionalism», treatment and «care», *at the same time*.

7.2.2. The nursing home as professionalized and personalized

Relating to the notion of the institution as bureaucratized is the more practically oriented notion of «professionalization»[1]. Professionalization, in

---

[1] «Professionalization» will be understood as a general term relating to the processes of structure, efficiency and management, rather than as is often the case in a Norwegian context, to the traits of and relationships between specific professional groups. Professional groups are part of the concept of «professionalization», in my understanding, but not exclusive to it. In Norwegian, I am referring to the process of «profesjonalisering» rather than «profesesjoner».

this context, relates again, like bureaucracy, to the idea of management control (or managerialism) and to demands of efficiency. At the same time, professionalization is neutral, independent of the specific agents. As such, professionalization, moving from a conceptual to a practical level, can be dichotomized by «personalized care»: that is the organization and implementation of work dependent on the local context, those who perform and those who are performed on, governed by initiative and expediency rather than rules.

Nursing homes are organized in particular ways, and more often than not follow the same organizational schematic. At the top are a leader and middle management primarily working with administrative and financial tasks. These positions tend to be occupied by registered nurses with some form of secondary education within «leadership» or «business». Institutional leaders do not generally work directly, perhaps not even indirectly, with residents. The size of nursing homes determines the size of the administrative corps, which in some instances also includes positions for personnel- and/or finance manager. These professional groups deal with the general aspects of the operation of the nursing home; finance, administration, commerce, and personnel, cut off from the everyday life of the units. The tasks they perform, and the specific positions defined for the performance of the tasks, are surprisingly similar from nursing home to nursing home, regardless of whether the nursing home reports to a commercial company, a non-profit organization, or a public entity.

In the units, the arena for staff-resident interaction, work is also professionalized. Not only are most positions filled by nationally or internationally recognized and validated professional groups like physicians, registered nurses and other categories of nurses (the latter more varied from country to country), but these groups, especially the positionally dominant registered nurses, serve specific functions within nursing homes. These functions, abstract (leadership, level of responsibility, level of manual labor) or specific (giving intravenous therapy, changing diapers, the administration of medicine), are largely monopolized by the respective professional groups. Registered nurses are allocated a certain domain of tasks and functions (leadership, giving intravenous therapy, the administration of medicine, for instance), primarily performed by them. The specific tasks allocated to registered nurses might, to some extent, overlap with those of assisting nurses (the administration of medicine for example), while their respective functions (primarily that of leadership and oversight, and organization and performance of resident care, respectively) are usually held separate. The tasks of assisting nurses might overlap with those of assistants, even more so than between registered nurses and assisting nurses, while their respective functions are somewhat different (primarily in the form of *organization* of resident care being made exclusively by assisting nurses). At most nursing homes the specific tasks performed by assisting nurses and assistants will be similar, while the responsibility of delegating them will not. The boundaries between the professional groups, and the degree of overlap between them, will vary (sometimes considerably) depending on the nursing home, perhaps most notably regarding registered nurses' involvement in assisting nurses' and assistants' domains. Internally, in each respective nursing home the boundaries and the degree of overlap are known and maintained.

The boundaries between the professional groups, spoken and unspoken, are seldom formalized in the form of written procedures. A formalized division of tasks is not necessary, as the division is known and practiced by all. In this sense, each professional group has its own methods, ideals and functions. While the division and boundaries between the respective groups are known and practiced on a daily basis, it is also presumed that other professional categories not included cannot replace those included. Other professional groups are excluded by default: residents of nursing homes *should* be cared for by registered and other nurses, they are the correct professional groups for the nursing home. These groups cannot simply be replaced by others (physical therapists, for instance). As such, professionalization is not strictly about formal competence per se, but rather about a peculiar competence relevant for *the nursing home.*

As mentioned, a significant segment of caring staff in nursing homes- categorized as assistants, have no formal education. Even though they comprise a central component of nursing homes, when considering their sheer numbers and tasks performed, they are considered less important than the professional groups in the sense that they are left with the tasks that do not fit with the ideal tasks for the professionals. This is no more evident than at morning report meetings which generally center on the tasks that have to be performed by registered nurses (and physicians, if present), and senior assisting nurses, before assistants are delegated their work. Assistant are, to be blunt, delegated whatever is left. As such, it is implied that the role of the assistants is not considered ideal; they are employed because of lack of nurses or because of a financial necessity.

Consequently, assistants are often encouraged to seek education as assisting nurses, since assisting nurses are encouraged to become registered nurses. Formal education, in other words, equals formal (position and salary[2], for instance) and informal (social capital, for instance) prestige, manifesting the «correctness» of the respective professional groups, including some, excluding others. As such, the function of assistants can be viewed as an exception to the general rule of professionalization, while, at the same time, confirming it: they do not fit into the ideal of professionalization and managerialism, but are simply a necessity.

The professionalization of nursing homes is also apparent in the (perhaps increasing) amount of administrative tasks, primarily in the form of documentation procedures, both in the central administration and in the everyday life of the units. While the general division of labor is not formalized in written procedures, caring staff vehemently assert that there is no shortage of documentation tasks they have to perform themselves. While the general regimes of reporting and accountability for Norwegian nursing homes have been pointed out earlier, often described as being in the tradition of «New Public Management» (Ingstad 2010), attention should also be given to connected regimes and routines at the micro-level, the units. The arena of direct person-to-person care is, in the experience of those who perform them, increasingly being dominated by tasks connected to reporting, measuring and documenting (Ibid.), and is certainly being perceived as such by caring staff (Jacobsen 2005). Although this is apparent for all professional groups, the amount of time spent on documenting seems to be proportional to the level of formal education. For unit leaders and some assistant unit leaders (there is more variation for the latter), a majority of time, if not all their time, is spent on administration and documentation. A large portion of this time is spent on the complex task of maintaining the shift plan. Especially assisting nurses with long experience from the nursing home sector are quick to point out the ever-increasing burden of responsibilities not connected to the care of residents, both for assisting nurses and others, seeing an increase in documentation for

---

2   The differences in salary between the professional groups (registered nurses – assisting nurses – assistants) are generally considered to be small in Norway compared to other countries, especially between registered nurses and assisting nurses. Also the difference in salary between the specialized (hospitals, for instance) and generalized (nursing homes, for instance) health sector is considered to be small in Norway.

registered nurses, for example, as also affecting them. The emphasis on administrative tasks and documentation is presented as detrimental to their «real» work: spending time in direct contact with residents. Registered nurses in particular (the assisting unit leader most of all) and assisting nurses constantly change between tasks connected to resident interaction and administration, making the measurement of the scope of documentation and administration difficult. Based on their own testimonies, however, both groups experience that the level of reporting and administration is not only too extensive, but also that is has increased.

Professionalization is, in practice, contrasted to what can be described as an ethos of «personalized care», that is, that which opposes regimes, hierarchies and procedures created by others than those who perform them. While the idea and ideal of professionalization can be said to be connected to an anonymous demand for effectiveness, the ethos of personalized care is connected to intimate and local knowledge. The notion of the nursing home as a professionalized arena of work is, then, opposed in nuanced and complex ways in nursing homes. Elsewhere, it has been pointed out that an anti-bureaucratic sentiment arises at the level of caring staff because the work that needs to be performed is inherently anti-bureaucratic (Jacobsen 2004). These attributes of what caring staff do, combined with the outside pressure of efficiency and streamlining, result in a less hierarchical division of labor than that of the hospital (Ibid.). The hierarchy, perhaps adapted from hospitals, is recognizable also in nursing homes, but is simultaneously in conflict with the ethos of personalized care. In nursing homes, informal recognition and position in the units, for instance, is gained by *experience*, by the specific know-how of everyday work, and not exclusively by formal authority. Assisting nurses with years of experience, for instance, can oppose the registered nurse, directly at report meetings in the morning, and indirectly by doing the job «her way» in opposition to suggestions from the unit leader. Other, more inexperienced nurses and assistants might also be inclined to follow the lead of the experienced assisting nurse, not necessarily by openly opposing the unit leader, but by following examples from the experienced assisting nurse, or asking her advice. The registered nurse, on the other hand, benefits from the experience of assisting nurses, and allies herself with key staff, to solidify her position in the micro-cosmos of the units' work environment. The hierarchical division of labor is resisted because of the attempts, in the view of the caring staff, to bureaucratize and professionalize, and thereby alienate them from the values nearest to their practice: «personalized» and «person-to-person care». As such, the hierarchy at the nursing home can be contested, perhaps in contrast to the hospital.

7.2.3. The nursing home as medicalized and care-based

To be understood as connected to the process of professionalization, while not completely overlapping, nursing homes *can* also be understood as medicalized, that is; as having a proclivity towards emphasizing medical competence and treatment in nursing homes, thus mimicking priorities, functions and procedures of the hospital. Such an ideology is clearly, implicitly and explicitly (in official white papers, for instance) opposed and contrasted to an ideology of «care». Care in this context refers to the function and acts of providing comfort and familiarity to residents (as opposed to medical treatment of patients) in their home (as opposed to the institution).

Nursing homes are described in law and generally in official white papers as medical facilities offering their residents (or, in this case «patients») medical treatment when necessary. As mentioned previously, the historical development of nursing homes in Norway has seen changes in the emphasis of treatment of the elderly, which was particularly strong in the 70s and 80s, while somewhat nuanced in later decades, including also a stronger emphasis on the home and being home-like in official white papers (Hauge 2004, Stortingsmelding nr. 25 2006). Nursing homes must, as will be discussed, constantly and continuously relate to the ambiguous tension of treatment and life-extension on one side and care and «normality» (related to the normal everyday life of *the home*) on the other. As Hauge has demonstrated, nursing homes can be seen as representing an unclear mixture of public and private (2004), while I would like to add to such a tension an ambiguous and involved relationship between *treatment* and *non-treatment*, relating to but also slightly different from the previous tensions mentioned.

Nursing homes can be said to be medicalized institutions in the sense of sharing professional roles (primarily in the form of physician, registered nurse and assisting nurse), and their respective positions in relation to each other (physician > registered nurse > assisting nurse), with the hospital. Integrated into each of these professional categories is also their respective (and thus relational) positioning towards «medical competence». In the same way as the appropriateness of the respective professional categories and their relational position, their positioning towards medical competence is taken for granted. The medical expertise and competence of both the physician and the registered nurses is widely considered, both in terms of the healthcare sector and popular opinion, to be positioned as they are and as important and integrated features of nursing homes. The question in the political and scientific discourse revolves not around their place in nursing homes, but rather about how much coverage of the respective professional groups should be considered sufficient (see for instance Hofacker et al. 2010 and Førde et al. 2006). As such, the nursing home is, at least formally, a medical institution resembling the hospital.

The tension between medicalization and «care» unfolds on different levels: on an abstract level in the sense that staff have to position themselves according to whether the nursing home should, ultimately, be a treatment facility for the ill or a provider of a home; and on a concrete level in the sense of providing emotional and practical, or physical support. Nurses and physicians have to deal with these dilemmas on a daily basis, often also pressured by family members. The daily life of nursing homes' staff is filled with small and large decisions, decisions that are related to questions of the cost-benefit of giving a resident a strong medicine, while at the same time being related to the larger question of what level of care should be provided in nursing homes. Such an ambivalence is constant for caring staff: there are no simple, correct solutions, no correct answer, nor does the outcome of their decisions – what happened to the resident – necessarily provide answers or prepare them for the next decision. As such, the nursing home is not medicalized to the extent of the hospital, simply because it cannot be; medical treatment of residents is not an unequivocal solution to the puzzles they have to solve.

Following on from the work of Hauge, who demonstrated an unclear relationship between the public and the private sphere (2004), and of Jacobsen, who argued that nursing homes are torn between being a home and bureaucracy (2005), I will argue that nursing homes are dichotomized by the values of *treatment* and *care*, relating to but not completely overlapping the previously discussed tensions. Consequently, caring staff in nursing homes relate to a constant ambivalence, to which there are no ready-made solutions. While such a discussion will be revisited in detail later, how the nursing home should be understood, in relation to these dilemmas, should be given some thought.

McCloskey and Hoonaard have argued that nursing homes and hospitals should be viewed as adhering to distinct and separable logical systems resulting in «(...) *two distinct worlds, which, for the most part, operate independently according to their own cultures and standards*» (2007: 189). On the contrary, I will argue that the systems and their *«cultures»* should not be viewed as representing an opposing logic and ethos *in effect*, but as overlapping. While I can agree with McCloskey and Hoonard that the logical systems can be identified and that one part is dominant (the field of medicine, represented by hospitals, primarily embodied by physicians) and one part is dominated (the field of care, represented by nursing homes, embodied primarily by caring staff), they should not be considered as distinctively separated. Nursing homes adopt and mimic procedures, terminology and, to some extent, the function of hospitals. Nursing homes not only share the professional categorization of the hospital, but also its hierarchy, its organizational structure, and, in many ways, its ethos. Nursing homes can, therefore, be placed within the *«medical field»* (Larsen & Adamsen 2008: 758), rather than opposing it. The overlap or tension between the two sets of logic can be illustrated by the constant and complex relationship between treatment and non-treatment: nursing homes are caught between opposing logical systems. Within such a change in perspective, *dominance* and *power* acquire different meanings than those proposed by McCloskey and Hoonard. Power within this perspective is not simply a case of discourse (within the research literature, being represented by a dominant logic) nor of explicit execution of power (by the field of medicine over the field of care). Rather, power is an implicit influence of one ideology over the other, through the establishment of a prevailing doxa (which remains largely uncontested by those dominated) through the execution of symbolic violence. The difference is both subtle and significant.

7.2.4. The nursing home as betwixt and between

The essence of the nursing home, its doxa, is not easily grasped, adding to the problematic endeavor of generalizing over nursing homes. A core can be identified, but when deconstructed into related layers, tensions and even contradictions are found. The nursing home is ambiguous in its very being, filled with variation and contradictions, consequently pulling its staff in contrasting and opposing directions. Specific nursing homes cannot be placed at a precise place in an abstract spectrum containing the ideas and values mentioned above, nor can caring staff choose one or the other. Rather, nursing homes are filled with lasting and constant tensions, from which there is no escape, producing changing outcomes. Life in nursing homes, more so than the general idea of the nursing home, is filled with dualities, dilemmas, ambivalences and opposing interests and ideas; for families, administration, governing bodies, and, especially caring staff.

Nor are the dichotomies presented necessarily in opposition to one another. The values of «bureaucracy» and «home», for instance, can be interpreted as omnipresent and overlapping in nursing homes, rather than strictly opposing values excluding one another. For example, based on a large workload and a feeling of being understaffed, caring staff can develop a need for *professionalism* in the form of organizing the workload and a distinct separation of duties, which might, perhaps paradoxically, enable them to give residents the feeling of living in *a home* (Jacobsen 2004). Dealing with these specific and abstract dilemmas on a daily basis, can also lead to experiencing a lack of direction in the work, as opposed to the more specific goals and tasks as hospitals, perhaps resulting in a more profound feeling of solidarity among the caring staff in nursing homes (Jacobsen 2005: 62-74).

As we shall return to in part three of the analysis, the tensions, for which there are no ready-made solutions, form the basis of *a fundamental uncertainty*, from which the development of local patterns of practice becomes an *absolute necessity*, ultimately taking the form of distinguishable, locally shared and functional sets of *institutional practice*. The institutional practice is developed and implemented not only because *it can*, because of the ambiguous nature of the work, but also because *it has to*; the ambiguous nature of the work calls for ways of systematizing knowledge and practice, not formally, but through the daily activities and choices in the units. Such a necessity is emphasized by three pivotal aspects of everyday life in nursing homes, which will be discussed in the next two chapters: challenges in dealing with residents, challenges relating to level of staffing, and the forms and functions of rules and regulations.

7.3. Meeting a resident: ambivalence towards Maud

Nursing home residents do, as others, socialize, form friendships, comraderies, oppose one another, and belong to groups or cliques. To a high degree, the socializing of residents at institutions can be based on affinities among residents who consider themselves equals in terms of social background or physical and cognitive skills (Bjelland 1982). Furthermore, the socializing of residents at institutions can be said to have an internal dynamic as well as being omnipresent for the residents, as the institution provides the setting for all or most of the social dynamics for the agents (Ågotnes 2005). As such, the agents develop and perform different roles, acknowledged within the microcosms of the institution, each attributed prestige and acknowledgment.

The way in which the residents are met, perceived, treated and categorized differently by staff, relates only in part to the role and position of the internal social dynamics among the residents. The perception of the caring staff towards a resident relates not as much to the social status of a resident as to how a resident fits with the caring staffs' interpretation and definition of their tasks and duties as caring staff: «how good a resident is to work with», in other words.

Maud

Maud is a resident at Acre Woods, where she has stayed for some time. She does not suffer from dementia or, seemingly, from any other cognitive impairments, but rather gives the impression of being very clear and present. She does, however, suffer from several physical ailments, making moving around and walking independently a great strain for her. She is dependent on care, especially during the morning and evening care routines. More than any resident in the unit, Maud is outspoken, constantly seeking conversational partners from residents, staff and visitors alike, a true extrovert. She has taken a role as a leader among residents, especially for the residents who usually sit in the small common room. Her seat in the small common room is seldom empty during the day, from about 8.30 until approximately 20.00. If it is empty, it is never occupied by anyone else. Maud's position as a prominent figure among the residents comes perhaps primarily from her energy and outspokenness, clearly surpassing that of her co-residents, who are often tired and lacking in energy. She is also extremely curious, always asking and always keeping tabs on other residents and visitors. She is seated so as to have a good overview of everyone entering the unit, usually stopping visitors and staff passing by. She has, through her constant conversations and her physical position, gathered great amounts of knowledge about residents, staff and visitors alike, which she often will refer to. In general, the staff have an ambivalent relationship to Maud; while enjoying conversing with a resident about more than the residents' needs, the caring staff members can also find her curiosity overwhelming.

After a meeting with the leaders of the unit, the physician is doing his rounds, visiting specific residents based on information from the meeting. Meanwhile, Maud is talking to one of the cleaners, a favorite conversational partner of Maud, about a television show that aired last night. When the physician is about to walk past the small common room, Maud stops him and waves him close: *Listen here. I´m having trouble with my breath. It´s really heavy. Can you help?* Maud has changed her tone of voice and facial expression considerably from talking to the cleaner: now a much sorrier version of her former self. The physician talks to her for a while, asking a couple of questions before saying they have to wait and see how her state develops for a couple of days before doing anything. Later, at lunch in the nurse's station, several of the caring staff raise the issue of Maud and her ailments, which Maud has expressed to them as well. One of them presents her as a *complainer* who dramatizes too much. Another nods in agreement and mentions other similar instances with Maud.

The next day, at breakfast time, Maud voices her dissatisfaction to me. She tells me that she is not feeling well at all and that she wishes to see the physician: *I´ve been unwell for several days now, and I don´t know what it is. I´m not getting proper help either.* Later, after asking for the physician several times through various caring staff, an assisting nurse calls for him, *even though it´s not his day*, she tells Maud. The physician arrives, talks to Maud for a short while, and proceeds to discuss «the case of Maud» with two assisting nurses and a registered nurse. One of the assisting nurses explains to the physician how difficult she finds dealing with Maud: *She really acts*[3] *a lot, making herself vulnerable. I don´t think there is much wrong with her. If so, it´s mainly psychological.* The physician gives the impression of sympathizing with the assisting nurse and says there is nothing he can do with regard to medication for her at this stage. He further explains that he has talked to Maud about this, and explained the situation to her. All of them, standing in the hallway close to the small common room, keep their voices down, cognizant of Maud trying to listen in on their conversation. After a suggestion from the registered nurse, to which the physician concurs, they decide to give Maud her regular dinner medication earlier, hopefully with the

---

3   «Act» is translated from the Norwegian «spiller», which, in this context, refers to the practice of exaggeration when presenting oneself.

effect of *settling her nerves*. Right after the conversation, I am stopped by Maud again, who is noticeably agitated: *Have you ever been to your doctor and just been told that there is nothing to do? What is that? I think I need to speak to my specialist. He is a very prominent man, you know. He always listens to me.*

Maud recovered and quickly returned to her normal self. Soon after, Maud went on a diet, with the expected effect of making her more mobile and helping her breathing. It was my understanding that the diet was planned and executed after a mutual agreement between Maud, her daughter, the physician and the assisting unit leader. After about a week on the diet, Maud addressed the issue, as she had done often in the days before. She seemed upset in part because the diet did not have the wanted effect, in part because she did not like the regimen. I listened to her, nodding in sympathy, trying not to say anything that could be understood as siding either with the caring staff or Maud. Still, Maud wanted more from me: *But, really, how do you think it is best to lose weight?* Diplomatically, I answered that I believed the only ways to lose weight was either to eat less or eat healthier food than before, so that the total calorie intake decreased. She shook her head: *But, dearest, I only eat four pieces of bread each day! And I don't eat any sugar! I was given some candy the other day, but I just gave it away. Besides, my daughter tells me that I get far too little for breakfast.* The next day, at the morning report meeting, Maud and her diet were discussed extensively. To my understanding, Maud's diet had been a source of much attention and frustration during the previous days, which now came to the surface. An assisting nurse first raised the subject by saying that it was difficult to help Maud because she *keeps hiding food in her room, which she eats all day.* In addition, Maud had been asking caring staff not directly involved with the diet to buy food for her, the assisting nurse adds. Another assisting nurse concurs by nodding. *We need to be careful in trusting her, because she has her own agenda,* a third assisting nurse says.

Two days later, Maud is still discussed at the report meeting. The unit leader raises the issue by explaining that Maud, somehow, has received information about the weight of another resident (a resident who is on a similar diet to Maud's). Maud has, in discussions with staff, been arguing for a change in her diet, referring to the other resident's weight, according to the unit leader. *This* (referring to the giving of personal information about one resident to another) *is a clear breach of the confidentiality agreement and cannot happen again,* the leader says, in a sterner tone of voice than usual. The staff remain silent for a little while, before an assisting nurse continues. She agrees with the leader but also says that helping Maud is difficult, because Maud wants to lose weight but at the same time is *cheating*. Another assisting nurse concurs, saying that Maud eats food in her room when no one is around: *I've found chocolate paper by her bed several times*, and that she *pits the caring staff against one another by asking for favors and then telling other staff how that one usually does it, and pressuring them to do the same.* The meeting is concluded by the assisting unit leader saying that the best way forward is to have a meeting after the weekend with Maud and her family, where she (the assisting unit leader) can explain that they want to help, but that they cannot do it properly if Maud does not want it herself.

The next day, the forthcoming meeting is raised again by the assisting unit leader. She asks for input from all staff members, for her to be as prepared as possible. An assisting nurse says that she found chocolate in Maud's room, which Maud had said that she had given away. Two other assisting nurses laugh, one of them says *typical*. An assistant says that Maud *complains* a lot to her daughter, with the intention of her daughter raising the subject with the staff. A registered nurse weighs in: *We need to be careful with the information we give her and about what she says to us. She filters what she likes and does not, so it is difficult to trust everything.*

One week later, four days after the meeting with Maud and her family, the issue of Maud and her diet resurfaced again at the report meeting, after being noticeably absent for several days. Towards the end of the report meeting, a registered nurse brought up Maud's diet as a side note to a discussion about the day's activities. The registered nurse said that Maud keeps asking for extra food, especially waffles in the activity center. Several other staff members concurred, mentioning examples when Maud has asked for refills of her agreed upon portion. An assisting nurse shook her head in disapproval. The assisting nurse concludes the matter by saying that they cannot use too much time babysitting Maud: *She needs to be able to take responsibility for herself.* I perceived the mood to be changing among the caring staff, almost to the point of resigning their previous effort.

Two weeks later Maud and her behavior towards the staff are raised again at the report meeting. In the preceding two weeks, both the staff and Maud have talked less about the diet. To my knowledge, the diet has gradually been phased down in the preceding weeks. The staff talk about their approach to Maud in more general terms than before. An assisting nurse says that she finds Maud difficult to deal with: *But not only for us, also for visitors who are questioned every day when they walk past.* The unit leader replies: *Well, in general we can do two things; we can either dismiss her if we feel she is taking it too far* (referring to Maud's sharing and asking about private information), *or we can play along. But it is important to be professional and not to be personal.* The assisting unit leader weighs in, to support the leader's point: *For instance, it has come to my attention that Maud has the private phone number of some of the nurses, and calls them privately. That is not ok. We need to separate private time and the job, and should not talk to them in our leisure time.*

«Hardship and toil» in the nursing home

Basically, we have to do everything: care, wash, clean, tidy up, make the food and fix things. You don't really have time for a calm moment. And then the day is over, just like that. Before, we were much more specialized. The different duties were divided between us, and we worked more on certain things and not with everything. In many ways I liked that better. (Experienced assisting nurse, Coruscant)

An integrated part of the doxa of the nursing home is a notion of the hardship of working there, a notion which in the following will be broken down into its respective components and analyzed through empirical data from our nursing homes. It will be argued that staffing levels and challenges connected to relating to *the nursing home resident*, in combination with a structural framework facilitating institutional autonomy, create a social world within which what is done and how it is done *need to be developed*.

8.1. Working in a nursing home

Set against the more descriptive overview of our nursing homes given in Chapter 3, we will now move towards two related and particularly important aspects of our nursing homes: the workload for caring staff connected to levels of staffing, and the characteristics of *the nursing home resident*. Perceptions about workload and residents are formative identity markers for the collective of caring staff, which together allude to the hardship or the toil of working in nursing homes as caring staff.

The hardship and toil of caring staff members influence not only the organization of work, but also how residents are perceived and, ultimately, met and treated in nursing homes. Caring staff members consider, for instance, lengthy conversations with residents a luxury they can ill afford in the hectic schedule of everyday life. Talking to residents *for the sake of talking*, in addition to other «soft» aspects of care, such as holding the hand of an unsettled resident or going for a walk outside, are not the first priority in our nursing homes. The caring staff convey that they simply have too much that has to be done during their respective shifts, with too many residents. In this way, doing more than what is considered absolutely necessary, in accordance with the basic needs of the residents and the primary objectives of the staff, is not prioritized, a sentiment also expressed elsewhere, stressing that there is little time for «chatting» and tending to the social needs of residents (Jacobsen 2005). This is not to say that caring staff do not wish to cater to the psychosocial well-being of their residents, nor that they do not see the need for it, but rather that they deem it beyond their individual and collective capacity. Consequently, having a lengthy, casual conversation with a resident is considered an interruption from what one really is supposed to do, almost to the point of being a private break, like having a cup of coffee in the nurses' station. The total amount of work that has to be performed during a shift can be seen as a constant zero-sum game: X amount of residents need to be given the morning care routine by Y amount of caring staff members, in addition to meals, toilet visits and so on. If so much as one staff member deviates from the collective plan of ensuring the fulfillment of these tasks, more needs to be done by others. From the perspectives of the caring staff, they have no choice. They have to relate to the fact that the home is inadequately staffed, and that they have too many tasks with too many residents in too little time, resulting in a sense of community in the form of a *«fellowship of poverty and toil»*, as discussed by Jacobsen:

> *«That one manages to get the work done despite a poverty of economic and personnel resources was an important and recurring theme among the nursing home staff. These workers stressed that they worked more than their health, strength and energy allowed. In other words, the work got done against all odds. Given the fact that maximum efforts were needed from each and every staff member on every work shift in order to perform the most needed tasks one should by definition have nothing more to give after the basic care was provided. Even the small extra burden of work carried out by the rest of the personnel when a particular worker performed less than his or her share was experienced as a threat to the delicate balance between the labor force and the tasks to be performed.» (2005: 73)*

As such, caring staff not only have to relate to the idea of not having sufficient time to cater to all the needs of the residents, but also adapt to and, to a certain extent, *enforce* such an idea. Furthermore, by adopting and enforcing the ideas of what can, needs to and should be done, caring staff also enhance and reproduce such ideas; the care of residents' psychosocial needs is beyond the realm of what could be done.

Relating to the prevalent doxa of the hardship of the caring staff is, as mentioned, the notion of the poor condition of today's nursing home resident, as briefly presented. She (a majority are female) is presented by popular opinion, policy documents, research *and caring staff* as old, frail, and in constant need of a variety of care. This sentiment is supported by the high threshold of admittance to nursing homes; potential residents must not only be in need of extensive, varying care to gain admittance, but must also wait before being admitted, and, for a great majority, must try other forms of public eldercare before admittance.

These doxic representations are related; residents are frail and demand a large amount of attention, while the number of caring staff is considered disproportional measured against the amount of challenges relating to the residents. In the following, the characteristics and composition of both nursing home residents and the level of staffing for caring staff will be analyzed. The level of staffing for caring staff will be discussed in relation to the effects and consequences for the organization of the daily work routines, which ultimately affects how residents are met and cared for. The number and composition of caring staff members, in other words, are relational to the ebb and flow of everyday life in nursing homes. In a previously cited study, Kayser-Jones (et al. 1989) found that too few caring staff members overall[1] and too few formally trained nursing staff[2] were the most influential of all relevant factors for the occurrence of hospitalizations that could and should have been avoided. As such, the priorities caring staff have to make relational to who and how many they are, are relevant not only for the general, everyday approaches to residents, but also influential for decisions on hospitalizations.

---

1   Exemplified by a caring staff member helping to feed 5-6 residents simultaneously, leaving her incapable of monitoring fluid intake, which led to a resident being hospitalized for dehydration.
2   Illustrated by the inability to administer intravenous therapy even when available.

8.2. The nursing home resident revisited

While nursing home populations are typically presented (by those working with them and those analyzing them) as collective groups given certain characteristics, being «old and frail» or representing a «high level of acuity», for instance, variation between residents is easily missed. A meeting with three nursing home residents might illustrate this point, while presenting a notion of the general obstacles caring staff have to relate to, every day, in their meetings with a complex and dependent «group» of residents.

Acre Woods, after dinner, on a weekday. As usual, the period right after dinner was noticeably calm in the unit, compared to any other time during the day-shift. A majority of the residents had returned to their rooms for an after-dinner nap, while others sat in chairs or wheelchairs in the common rooms dozing off. In the large common room, only three residents still sat at the large dining table, while caring staff finished with the task of cleaning up. Leif, Alexandra and Constance sat at their usual places, some distance from each other, but still within speaking range. Alexandra was still eating while Leif and Constance simply sat in peace looking out into thin air, or so it seemed. There were no caring staff present to talk to, nor did they talk amongst themselves. In total, they formed an unlikely group. Alexandra (see also Chapter 6.2.), cognitively lucid, had walked into the common room by herself with the specific aim of getting food. Leif, suffering from advanced dementia and with severely slurred speech was helped to his seat by the staff. Constance (see also Chapter 8.4.), also suffering from dementia but with good communication skills, had wandered into the common room by herself, seemingly disoriented and sitting down randomly. They seemed, to me, to be lonely together, unable to communicate amongst themselves, and having no one else around.

Of the three residents, Leif was the only one who would usually sit at the large table, more often than not alone, often making comments to no one in particular. Alexandra usually stayed in her room, and was only seen or heard in the common room during mealtimes or shortly before and after. Constance was often in the common room, but seldom for consecutive periods of time, as she liked to move around, walking by herself. She seldom sat still for more than five minutes. I sat down with the three, after asking about how they had enjoyed dinner. Constance and Alexandra particularly gave the impression of welcoming the company, while Leif was indifferent. Sitting down and talking to the three seemed like the sensible thing to do for me, as the common room was desolate and quiet, not offering any impulses for these three who did not appear to be tired at all, as opposed to the rest of the residents in the unit.

Getting a conversation started proved, however, extremely difficult, as the three responded differently, if at all. After a while, I gave up, a bit frustrated at my inability to be sociable with all three. Instead, I suggested that I could read the newspaper, which I proceeded to do. I read the highlights of some of the news bulletins and commented in between. This small exercise also proved difficult, as I did not understand how much I should explain and contextualize regarding the respective headlines. Knowing the three residents in advance only complicated it; I knew that Alexandra was well-informed on current events, and could communicate effortlessly, even though she seldom chose to do so. Constance, on the other hand, was more difficult to communicate with; she spoke fluently but did not always respond as one would expect, her mind drifting off. Leif posed different obstacles altogether; he would often make a comment on his own accord or respond when talked to, but was difficult to apprehend as his speech was slurred and mumbled. Consequently, it was hard to know what he apprehended. While I read the newspaper, the three residents' reactions and comments mirrored my impression of them. Alexandra made few, but astute and well-informed comments. Constance paid close attention to what was being said and commented on everything, to the irritation of Leif, but was seldom to the point, while Leif did not appear to be paying attention, and made some comments which I interpreted to be about an entirely different subject (relating to fishing). It seemed to me that I had done a decent job of informing and communicating with Alexandra, while what I did and how I did it was not appropriate for Constance and Leif. Had I done it differently, by taking more time and explaining in a more detailed manner, Constance and perhaps also Leif might have benefitted more, although I am uncertain about Leif. However, Alexandra would perhaps have found it degrading, as if talking to a child.

The portrayal of the nursing home resident as old, frail and dependent is omnipotent among caring staff members. Residents are presented as utterly dependent on various forms of assistance, *or else they would not be here*. The challenges for residents are, as illustrated by Alexandra, Leif and Constance, varied and complex; *the nursing home resident* is afflicted with various forms or degrees of dementia often in combination with various forms and degrees of a multitude of physical ailments.

8.2.1. The nursing home resident of today and yesterday

They don´t arrive here with their suitcase in hand anymore (Unit leader)

A brief description of resident characteristics was given in Chapter 3, highlighting age, dementia and ADL-functions. Comparing these characteristics to a similar sample, the question of whether nursing home residents are older and frailer than before will be asked. The short answer is yes and possibly.

Comparable data were gathered for a similar sample (four large and five small nursing homes in Norway) in 1980 (Slagsvold 1986), while a smaller study providing data on residents' age was conducted in 1999 (Hauge 2004). Comparing current data on resident characteristics with the data from 1980 can be beneficial as the data are based on a similar sample and use the same categories of resident characteristics[3]. However, both samples are small, and the data are only for 1980 and 2013/2014, aside from age in 1999. The respective data should therefore be viewed as snapshots typical of a specific period rather than representing a generalizable development from the past until present. In line with the doxic representations of today's nursing home resident, the nursing home population has aged considerably in a relatively short time span: from 81.9 years (Slagsvold 1986), to 86,7 years (Hauge 2004), to 89.2 years (within our sample), on average. Today's nursing home resident *is* older than yesterday's.

But is she necessarily frailer? Looking both at figures for general and specified ADL-measures, it seems that conclusions on the development of resident frailty are harder to make. The average number of residents with dementia and suffering from incontinence has risen considerably: from 21 percent to 71 percent for dementia, and from 43 percent to 79 percent for incontinence. However, when looking at average numbers for two of the activities of daily living, the tendency is contradictory: 33 percent of residents in 1980 were considered to be able to «eat individually» in contrast to 84 percent in our sample. 29 percent of residents in 1980 were considered to be able to «walk independently», in contrast to 50 percent in our sample. Other activities of daily living produced different outcomes altogether: 26 percent of residents in 1980 were considered to be able to

---

3   The categories used (see Chapter 3) were partly open to interpretation from the respondents. As the characteristics are not completely operationalized in the former study, inclusion of residents into categories such as «incontinence», might be based on differing perceptions from the respondents.

«wash themselves independently», in contrast to only 6 percent in our sample, while 24 percent of residents in 1980 were considered to be able to «dress themselves independently», in contrast to only 8 percent in our sample.

The seemingly paradoxical variation can perhaps be explained by differences in interpretation of the respective categories. Alternatively, some of the variation can be ascribed to a change in the criteria of admission to nursing homes, signaling, perhaps, an increased emphasis on the diagnosis of dementia rather than physical ailments. Nursing home residents of today certainly have a high prevalence of dementia (higher also than yesterday's residents), while these residents may or may not have severe physical ailments in addition to dementia. Washing and dressing independently can be interpreted as activities relatively unrelated to cognitive awareness, while eating independently might be contrary, thus perhaps explaining the confounding differences between the two samples. In an ethnographic study taking place in 1990 in a Norwegian nursing home, the relatively high number of residents dependent on wheel-chairs (62 percent) was emphasized (Jacobsen 2005), indicating a level of physical frailty similar to that of our sample. In the cited study, 59 percent of residents were reported to be diagnosed with dementia, contrary to such a hypothesis. A third interpretation of this apparent paradox is a potential change in the general practice of nursing homes. For the two ADL measures where present nursing home residents scored higher, eating and walking, caring staff can potentially *facilitate* resident autonomy. Meals, for instance, can be prepared and presented in such a way that residents can eat individually, by grinding the food (for residents with bad teeth), presenting the cutlery correctly (by the functional arm for a resident with a paralyzed arm), or adjusting a food tray high enough (for a resident in a wheelchair), as seen done every day, albeit to a varying degree, in our nursing homes. Similarly, caring staff can act as facilitators so that residents can walk more freely, especially by individualizing aides such as walking frames. For the two ADL measures where present nursing home residents scored significantly lower than the sample from 1980, washing and dressing, the possibility for caring staff to facilitate resident autonomy is more limited. Clothes and washing remedies can be presented in advance, but if residents are physically unable to move into the bathtub or unable to bend down, they will need assistance in performing the activities regardless of facilitation.

If this hypothesis holds true, two implications can be drawn. Current caring staff seem to be more finely attuned to the *facilitation of resident independency* than caring staff in the past. Secondly, nursing home residents are more frail and dependent, regardless of caring staff efforts. These two implications might also be connected: if residents are less independent now, caring staff *have to be* proficient in facilitating activities of daily living, not only for the benefit of the residents, but also for the workload of the staff. By preparing the meals and adjusting the cutlery individually, for instance, caring staff will not only cater to the residents' individual needs, but also save time if the alternative is to feed residents by hand, as is often the case. However, the idea of the relative deterioration of nursing home residents' independency is contrasted by the number of bedridden residents: 26 percent in 1980 and 6 percent in the recent sample, adding to the contradicting characteristics of the two samples.

To summarize, today's nursing home resident can be considered old and frail. The forms of frailty, however, are difficult to measure and analyze when compared to yesterday's resident. Perhaps staff relate differently to residents today out of necessity; residents not only should but also must perform certain daily activities independently, when possible.

8.2.2. Variation of today's residents within the institution

As illustrated by the responses to the reading of the newspaper, today's nursing home residents should not be presented as a homogeneous group; they will vary within an institution and from institution to institution, and not only in time. The variation in residents adds to the difficulties of caring staff, not only by having a large total workload, but also residents with very different needs, adding to the effect of an already profound uncertainty among caring staff, to be discussed. Some residents, especially with diminished language and/or advanced dementia can, for instance, be difficult to understand and interpret:

> Acre Woods, my first day in *the other unit*, Tuesday early afternoon, between lunch and dinner. I have just concluded my initial talk with the unit leader, and decide to walk around the unit for a couple of hours. I enter the large common area (identical to that of *the unit*). There are three tables in the common room, one large dining table, and two smaller coffee tables. The tables are placed with some distance between each, giving their respective occupants relative privacy. Three residents are sitting at the large table. They do not appear to be sitting together, but rather randomly placed at some distance from each other. They do not communicate. Without knowing quite why, I get the impression that they have remained here since breakfast, while the rest

of the residents who had been sitting there have gone to their rooms. Two other residents are sitting at a small table at the end of the room. A caring staff member (whom I do not know) is sitting with them, talking sporadically, while another is about to leave. I sit down at the large table between two of the residents. One of the residents at the table is sitting leaned backwards in her wheelchair with her eyes closed. I think she is sleeping. The second resident is awake, also in a wheelchair, and is sitting leaning forward with her head awkwardly low and her face turned away from me. Her body is twisted, especially her left arm and hand, from what I assume is arthritis. She seems very fragile and immobile. The third resident, Ida, is awake and appears to be attentive. She acknowledges me with a nod. Ida is nicely dressed and has a vigilant and clear gaze. She, as opposed to the other two residents, has good posture, her back straight and knees together. My initial impression of her is of a nice and «correct» woman. My attention is directed towards her, partly because she acknowledges my presence, partly because it seems like an easier task to communicate with her compared to the others. She keeps her gaze on me, as an invitation to make contact, or so I perceive it. I change my stance so as to address her more easily.

Me: *So, finished with breakfast?*

Ida: *Yes, it was lovely.*

Me: *I'm Gudmund and I've come from the university college. I'm here as part of a research project, so I'm visiting nursing homes to learn how it is here.*

Ida: *Oh, how exciting! I have a son who is a teacher, so I know about that, yes.*

Ida's dialect is a distinguished one, her tone of voice calm and correct. She talks fluently, confidently, and does not struggle to find the words. She seems comfortable. We talk for about five minutes about the university college and about her son. Meanwhile she is pleasant company, and seems to have a good understanding of what is going on.

Me: *So, what school does your son teach at?*

Ida: *What on earth do you mean? There is only one school here in Tromsø!*[4]

---

4   Naming a city far from our municipality, the name of which has been altered.

For the first time in the conversation she seems uncertain of herself. I am not sure if that is caused by confusion or by being surprised by my ignorance. Her gaze and movement indicate that something is out of place. So as not to unsettle her anymore, I politely end the conversation and thank her for the company. I leave the common room and go for a walk around the unit. About thirty minutes later, I return. The same residents are present, but they are seated differently. Ida now sits by a small coffee table in a corner of the room, together with three other residents, two of whom were seated with her earlier. They now sit closer together, within hearing range of one another. I join them. Ida nods towards me and smiles. I return the gesture, silently. Ida then leans in towards me and whispers, almost conspiratorially:

Ida: *I do not want to be rude and point, but that one there* (she carefully directs her gaze at a resident sitting next to her, who does not notice the gesture) *cannot do anything herself. She needs help with everything, poor thing.*

As to underscore her point, Ida gently shakes her head. She leans back for about five seconds, before leaning in again and continuing:

Ida: *The other one* (she nods lightly towards another resident) *is not present at all. And that one* (nods towards the last resident) *does not understand anything either.*

She lets out a small laugh and leans back again. When she continues, she remains like this, within hearing range of the other residents, but still directs her conversation towards me.

Ida: *Well, well. It is not nice to laugh, but I guess we all get a little bit cuckoo sometimes.*

Me: *Yes, I suppose so.* There is a 10 second pause before Ida continues.

Ida: *One thing I am wondering about, for example: I have been on this boat for ages now, and thought we were going to Oslo[5]. But what business do I have there?*

---

5   Another city far from our municipality. The name of the city has been altered.

She looks at me, quizzically, obviously unsure of herself. Her uncertainty is now noticeable, and a stark contrast to her previous, confident self. I interpret her uncertainty as a fundamental one; she seems genuinely unsure of her surroundings and her place in them, and might even be scared as a consequence.

Ida, lucid, present and vigilant, appears to be in control of herself and her surroundings. At first glance there is nothing about her indicating she needs to be cared for in a long-term caring institution. But appearances can be deceiving; Ida is lost at sea, but also lost in regard to familiarity; she cannot recognize her surroundings nor her place in them. As such, Ida does not seem to fit in with the stereotype of a nursing home resident: she is neither physically impaired nor does she appear to have cognitive impairments. She is confident and assertive, far from the idea of the frail nursing home resident. Ida, then, illustrates the heterogeneity of nursing home residents, a heterogeneity not necessarily in the form of having a diagnosis or not (which Ida had), or different diagnoses (a majority are diagnosed with Alzheimer's or dementia) but in the form of different everyday manifestations of a diagnosis or of frailty in general, implying various and different approaches from caring staff. Ida, as such, illustrates the difficulties of interpreting nursing home residents, as they adapt to their surroundings, have different needs, and express themselves in different and complex ways. Consequently, *relating* to residents of nursing homes can be challenging, difficult and frustrating, especially for caring staff. Relating to residents can be challenging because *their* challenges are varied, in form and severity, and also because residents can be difficult to interpret, understand and «read», like Ida.

8.2.3. Variation of today's residents between the institutions

Residents are not a homogeneous group. They vary considerably within a nursing home (or unit), in how physically dependent they are, in how they present themselves, in what they need, and in what they can or will give the impression of what they need, as seen with Ida. But does the total level of acuity of groups of residents vary considerably between nursing homes? Do some nursing homes have residents who are less frail than others? This question relates, of course, directly to institutional variations in hospitalization. If the answer is clearly «yes», we can end our investigation here.

Measuring levels of acuity, especially for a group of residents, is problematic and difficult. One aspect of nursing home life that might give some indication of how «well-functioning» residents are, is how active they are. When going from one nursing home to the next during the initial period of fieldwork, I was struck by how different the resident population of each nursing home appeared. Especially in two nursing homes, Durmstrang and Emerald Gardens, residents seemed to be far more physically mobile, more active in general and more vocal (to other residents and to staff), than in the other four nursing homes. While the level of mobility and activity of residents is difficult to measure, as are the *reasons* for the level of activity and mobility, some reflections regarding these questions can be raised. Residents at Durmstrang and Emerald Gardens might have been relatively more capable to start with, or, perhaps more probably, caring staff in these two small nursing homes had a more explicit approach towards facilitating mobility and activities with and by residents.

As for the first point, nursing home residents are admitted to a nursing home by the municipality through a specific municipal department, and not by the respective nursing homes, securing, supposedly, a relatively similar total nursing home population at each institution. It is difficult, however, to account for the accuracy of the intended even distribution among nursing homes, as neither the municipality nor the respective nursing homes grade or classify residents' functional abilities in any systematic form that could allude to the total level of acuity for each nursing home.

In addition to a potential organizational preselecting of residents, the resident population of the respective nursing homes can hypothetically differ based on socio-economic background, and thus be considered a pre-selection of population related to area of residence. As such, nursing home populations in the respective nursing homes could be analyzed based on their cumulative capital (economic, social and cultural), in accordance with the general assumption of the association between capital and health. To make such an analysis, however, one would need extensive access to residents' personal histories, both in the form of nursing home journals and interviews with residents and families (as many residents would not be able to provide information themselves). I did not have access to such information, nor the ethical approval for gathering it. Based on observational data, meanwhile, the composition of residents within our sample did not seem to be connected to the area in which the nursing homes were located.

As for the second point - the respective nursing homes' focus on and ability to facilitate resident mobility and activity - the two nursing homes with apparently more functional residents, Durmstrang and Emerald Gardens, did seem to have a more explicit approach than most other nursing homes, albeit in different ways. Emerald Gardens had a well-established and widely used activity center, used collectively by all residents at the nursing home. Additionally, caring staff at this nursing home seemed to spend more time on idle conversations with residents. The latter may not in itself be directly related to activation, but certainly contributes to a general atmosphere of inclusion and staff-resident communion. Emerald Gardens, as described in Chapter 9, also had a physical layout which contributes to interaction between residents and between residents and staff; it is centered around an accessible common room, providing indistinct boundaries between staff and residents. Durmstrang, meanwhile, did not excel in a similar way when it came to staff-resident interaction, or the activation and stimulation of residents. Whilst there was no activity center, the staff did spend more time than any other nursing home in finding individual activities for each resident. As such, it was the responsibility of the respective caring staff, rather than an activity worker, to engage the residents in specific and non-specific exercises and activities. This form of organization led to individual variations – some caring staff took these tasks more seriously than others – and variations between units. Although the efforts to activate residents at this nursing home at times exceeded that of other nursing homes, it still seems implausible to attribute the apparent high level of resident functionality to this practice.

It is extremely difficult to identify a causal relationship between the approaches of the nursing homes and the functional abilities of their residents. The complex relationship between approaches and functional ability is further complicated by the fact that all nursing homes have some variant of the approaches illustrated by the two mentioned nursing homes, although not as distinct. However, Durmstrang and Emerald Gardens *did* excel when it comes to facilitating activities for residents, to residents' uncontested benefit. A point that strengthens the assumption of the staff's approach, as opposed to pre-selection of resident population, as significant for overall functional ability, is the tendency of Galactic Manor to develop different, unit-specific approaches to resident-staff interaction, resulting in noticeably different levels of resident activity. Galactic Manor distributed its residents among the respective units in such a way that the total workload in each unit was as even as possible.

Nevertheless, the respective units developed different approaches towards their residents, as we shall see in more detail later.

A point not alluded to, but still of importance, is the level of the use of psychotropic drugs in nursing homes. It is commonly assumed that the relative widespread use of psychotropic drugs by nursing home residents, being administered to 75 percent of Norwegian nursing home residents suffering from dementia according to one source (Selbæk et al. 2007), can lead to more sedated residents, as might have been the case of Cate (Chapter 1.4). Hypothetically, differing practices in the administration of psychotropic drugs between nursing homes can lead to different overall levels of activity and *apparent* levels of acuity among the respective resident populations. As I did not have access to residents' medical journals, comparing nursing homes' practices in using psychotropic drugs is problematic, emphasized by the unwillingness of caring staff to discuss the subject[6]. The potentially differing practice in administering psychotropic drugs still stands out as an essential topic for further research, especially when considering the overall workload of caring staff in nursing homes, as alluded to in the introduction to this chapter. As such, the administration of psychotropic drugs, which in themselves can be considered drugs without absolute treatment regimens, and thus can be said to fall under or resemble the «*professional uncertainty principle*» discussed later, can be related to levels of staffing in nursing homes, to which we now shall turn. For the case of Cate, caring staff felt that she was not safe; she could easily fall again if her uneasiness and nervousness continued. Such a sentiment is, I believe, a direct result of level of staffing: Cate could not «be kept safe» because caring staff did not have time to monitor her constantly. In conclusion, residents in our nursing homes, are relatively homogeneous when comparing institutions. The differences observed between institutions regarding residents, appear to be connected to the approaches of staff, rather than a bias in the selection of residents.

8.3. The nursing home staff revisited

Small nursing home, name withheld. My first day at the nursing home had transpired relatively uneventfully. I had talked at length with the leader of the institution, been

---

6   In general, the topic of the administration of psychotropic drugs can be described as somewhat taboo in nursing homes.

given the «tour» of the nursing home, and explained my project in short to the respective staff. I spent the last two hours of the day in the kitchen/dining area of one of the units, where I have been introduced to some of the residents, as well as to the general routines in the unit. The day-shift was about to end, and I to leave, when, in a calm moment in the unit, I was approached by two assisting nurses with whom I have had the most contact. One of them stepped close to me and said, keeping her voice down but still within the hearing range of the other assisting nurse: *It is a good thing that you are here! It is a good thing that you have come to see how it really is!* I answered politely, though a bit unnerved by her impression of me changing the nursing home. I tried to explain that my main objective was to understand how caring staff worked and what drives them to do what they do, and not, ultimately to measure or evaluate nursing homes. The assisting nurse nodded, and continued enthusiastically: *You know what, it is difficult for us here. Especially during the weekends. We are simply too few. Not a single weekend-shift goes by without my having a bad conscience. I cannot do my job! I don't have a chance, it just doesn't add up. I know that others have it like this too, but it is difficult to talk about amongst ourselves.* She smiled, giving me the impression of her sharing a secret with me. The other assisting nurse nodded in agreement.

Staff in nursing homes present their everyday working life as hectic and hard. The level of staffing is generally considered to be low, too low, when compared to the amount and level of care needed by residents. As we have also seen, the main tasks and assignments of caring staff can be described as basic, in the sense of primarily being directed towards medical and everyday needs, rather than psychosocial needs related to the well-being of the residents.

In the following I will discuss the consequences of the level of staffing for the organization of work and for how caring staff relate to residents.

8.3.1. Level of staffing by numbers

The level of staffing for the hierarchically dominant professional groups, physicians and registered nurses, can generally be considered high when compared to the mentioned sample from 1980 (Slagsvold 1986). For the 1980 sample physician hours per week, per resident averaged 0.17 compared to 0.29 for our nursing homes. Based on these limited samples, today's nursing home physicians spend considerably more time *in total* in nursing homes than that of yesterday's[7]. Despite such a tendency, there are still considerable variations within each sample. Within our sample, as we have seen, physicians also vary regarding availability outside time spent at the nursing homes; paradoxically this is higher for physicians employed at the nursing homes and with close to full-time positions than those employed through the municipality and having fewer contracted hours.

Registered nurses' hours per week, per resident are also high for our sample compared to the 1980 sample: an average of 0.26 compared to an average of 0.13[8]. Staffing levels for registered nurses are, based on our limited sample, better today than they were yesterday. However, there are large variations within each sample; smaller nursing homes tend to have slightly better staffing levels for registered nurses (although there are large variations within the respective samples of «small» and «large» nursing homes as well). Although the average for today's sample is twice that of yesterday's, the nursing home with the highest level of registered nurses' staffing level from the 1980 sample is higher than the lowest from our sample.

The level of assisting nurses[9] has increased similarly to that of physicians and registered nurses, from the 1980 sample, an average of 0.17, to our sample, an average of 0.52. There are, in other words, more than three times more assisting nurses on average working in nursing homes today compared to the 1980 sample. It is perhaps surprising that this development mirrors that of registered nurses. Even more surprising, and contrary to the popular belief of fewer uneducated professional groups today, is a small increase in the number of assistants' hours per week, per resident, from 0.09 to 0.15.

The current level of staffing for the groups with the highest formal competence can be attributed to the general development of the nursing home sector during this time period, previously discussed. Based on the overview of current staffing levels, nursing homes today can indeed be described as institutions with high formal competence within the medical and healthcare field. The figures also indicate that nursing homes today are considerably better

---

7   This difference seems to be illustrative of a general national development, seeing an increase in physician hours per week, per resident from 0.27 in 2005 to 0.49 in 2014 when including all municipalities in Norway (www.helsenorge.no).

8   All these figures are based on intended figures for registered nurses' working hours, as opposed to actual figures for their working hours, which may vary as we have seen, as registered nurses are generally replaced by other professional groups when ill or on leave.

9   Including «omsorgsarbeidere» and «helsefagsarbeidere», professional titles not yet adopted in 1980.

staffed in total numbers. Also in an international context, the intended coverage of trained professionals in Norwegian nursing homes appears to be high (Harrington et al. 2012).

It should be noted, again, that these data (including the international comparison) are exclusively about *intended* levels of staff, based on nursing homes' budgetary definition of level of total and professionalized staffing. This does not necessarily correspond with reality. Sick leave and other forms of leave are abundant at our nursing homes and vacancies are typically either not filled or filled by professional groups with less formal competence than those occupying the vacant positions.

> Durmstrang, morning, weekday. I had been at the unit three times before, between two and four hours each time, and was beginning to feel familiar with the routines and «flow» there. This particular day, however, felt very different. There were only three caring staff members present, compared to the usual four, and one of them was new (she had just started her position at the nursing home). In addition to the new assisting nurse, the group leader and an experienced assisting nurse were present. As opposed to the other days I had spent at the unit, everything seemed to happen at a furious pace; there was little talking among the caring staff, except for giving instructions to the new assisting nurse, and even less talking between caring staff and residents. Breakfast, starting at about 8.30, (preparation for breakfast probably started before) lasted until approximately 9.50, much longer than usual, and was immediately followed by preparations for lunch. The caring staff, in other words, did not find time for anything besides preparing and serving the meals to the residents, during the first half of their shifts. To make matters worse, the group leader had to spend time in her office, making sure the following shifts were properly filled. For about an hour's time during breakfast, the experienced assisting nurse tended to the administration of medicine to the residents, and was solely occupied with this. At this point, the inexperienced assisting nurse was left alone with all the residents, not quite knowing what to do.

When considering the doxic representation of levels of staffing as presented by caring staff, and discussed initially in this chapter, we are left with a paradox; why do caring staff constantly and consistently focus on the hardships and toil connected to a feeling of being understaffed in relation to their workload? The answer, I believe, is to be found in part in the frailty of today's nursing home resident, in part in the organization and distribution of staffing (particularly at different periods of time, such as weekends, evenings, or holidays), which again must be seen in connection with financial incentives.

8.3.2. Effects and consequences of the level of staffing

It is just so busy here, that I sometimes wonder if it is even justifiable. We have three on day and two on evening, and especially in this unit, that is not enough. Is this really how we want to treat our elderly? Think about all that happens here, we have to care and make food and if something happens to a resident two of us need to see to her or him, and then there is no one left for the others! Especially here[10] that could lead to conflicts or even be dangerous. It is, at any rate, important to talk about these things, although I doubt it will get better.» (Assisting nurse, name of institution withheld)

Levels of staffing, in the sense of number and composition of caring staff compared to number of residents, will to a high degree determine how the day at the nursing home transpires. The level of staffing relates not only to what potentially could be done during a day or a shift, but also to how residents are treated, particularly with regard to the possibility of providing for more than their most basic needs. The level of staffing not only varies in time or between institutions, as seen above, but is also considerably different from day-, to evening- and night-shifts, and from weekdays to weekends. All nursing homes have a higher level of staffing on day-shifts on weekdays than any other shifts. The priority of having better staffing during the day on weekdays can be seen as a practical one, as most of the tasks relating to resident care occur during this time. Alternatively, one could argue that most of the tasks and activities are concentrated in the beginning of the day, *because* there are more staff in place at that time. Specific activities such as bingo or a quiz, typically take place before dinner, at around 12.00, further condensing the already hectic schedule for residents and staff during the day-shift. Other events and activities, such as physician visits, hairdressing and showers/baths, also occur within this period. As such, daytime in the nursing home, between approximately 8.00 and 15.00, resembles that of everyday life outside the nursing home. It is similar to the routine of children at school or the

---

10   «Here» refers to a dementia ward, implying that dementia wards can be particularly challenging in regard to the level of staffing.

average office worker; this period is hectic, follows a distinct, repeatable pattern, and is in contrast with the time afterwards, which is not routinized to the same extent and usually has a slower more changeable pace. This is how daytime in the nursing home can be experienced both by residents and caring staff. Nursing homes, then, strangely adapt to and mimic the norm of the outside world, without, in my opinion, the absolute need to do so. As we shall see, the contrary might also be the case.

Management of nursing home institutions can be said to have an incentive to prioritize day-shifts on weekdays over other shifts, as both evening-, night- and weekend-shifts (regardless of being day, evening or night) entail relatively large additions to the basic salary of the caring staff, additions that all institutions are obliged to give. All nursing home institutions, regardless of being private or public, are thus incentivized to prioritize certain shifts over others. Leadership at the nursing homes and, to a varying degree, the respective units, is pressured, from within and without, not to exceed a level of staffing considered «acceptable». The consideration of «acceptable» can be manipulated when it comes to filling short-term vacancies:

Informal conversation with a unit leader, Cloud House. After discussing the general features of the unit, the discussion turns towards the role of the unit leader. I ask about challenges in her daily work:

Unit leader: *Generally finance is a big challenge, especially when it comes to temporary positions.*

Me: *Can you expand, perhaps?*

Unit leader: *Well, for instance, if there are four on the day-shift and one is ill, we are really not supposed to cover that position, especially not from an agency[11]. In the end, it is the registered nurses who notice it the most, because they, then, cannot work on administration and other tasks and have to be a part of the everyday care.*

Me: *Is this common? Here and in general, you think?*

---

11   Agencies for temporary staff are used by nursing homes to varying degrees, and, in general, considered expensive.

Unit leader: *Very common. At least here. There is a lot of sickness. And that is not covered if there is a registered nurse attending. A lot of times it is not covered regardless, but that depends on who the two are[12] and who the potential temps are.* (Pause) *Basically, it all relates to cost.*

Returning to the relative lack of public staffing regulations and the subsequent autonomy of the respective institutions, discussed earlier, nursing homes can to a large degree prioritize staffing levels of the respective shifts independently. These priorities follow a distinct pattern: nursing homes prioritize day-shifts on weekdays, because they can, because they benefit from it, and because their organization, specifically the distribution of tasks between day- and evening-shift, facilitates such a prioritization.

As such, one could argue that caring staffs' experience of work as toil on evening-, night- and weekend-shifts, is connected to a perception of being under-staffed in relation to the number and caring needs of residents, and is self-inflicted by the institutions. In my opinion, the financial incentives weigh more heavily when organizing the shifts than the needs of residents during different time periods of the day. The argument for the necessity of having more caring staff in place during day-shifts solely based on the needs of the residents is challenged by the relatively low level of staffing during weekend day-shifts. During Saturday day-shift, for instance, residents will have the same or similar needs and will constitute the same or similar total workload for caring staff, as for day-shifts during weekdays (besides the self-afflicted added burden of organizing tasks and activities on weekdays), but are staffed differently. A similar point was made by Jacobsen (2005), stressing the relative similarities in total workload on the day-shift on weekends as that of working days, while having less personnel coverage (although not finding a similar discrepancy on evening-shifts).

Two separate examples, one episode and one excerpt of a day, can illustrate how the ebb and flow of daily activities for caring staff are connected to the level of staffing. It should be noted that both of these examples are from the same unit at Acre Woods, about one month apart, and involve many of the same residents and some of the same staff members.

---

12   Referring to the two caring staff members (not registered nurses) «left», and whether or not they are considered to be experienced or not.

Morning around 9.00, Acre Woods, weekday. Standing in the hallway observing the staff and residents during the busy morning routines, this morning struck me as particularly hectic. Most of the residents were eating breakfast already, either in the large common room or in their rooms. Maud was the only resident in the small common room, eating and trying to catch the attention of the caring staff organizing food on two large trollies just across from her. The respective staff members were quick to put whatever they needed on their trays and move on, towards the main common room or the room of a resident, not paying much attention to Maud. Shortly thereafter another staff member would replace the one that just left, to prepare her tray and then move on. Next to the two trollies, a registered nurse and an assisting nurse (with a course in medicine administration) were busy organizing the morning medicine. One of them, the registered nurse, would find the correct medicine, double check with the journals, while the assisting nurse would give it to its recipient. All the caring staff worked hard and worked swiftly, not pausing, not discussing and not deliberating about what they were supposed to do. They did not converse amongst themselves, besides the exchange of pleasantries, but sporadically took time to talk to a resident, wishing a good morning or asking what the resident would prefer to drink. At one point, an assisting nurse talked to Cate about a visit she was supposed to get later, before asking what kind of milk she would prefer. Cate did not reply to the question, as often happened, but another assisting nurse said that she prefers sour milk.

The individual and collective movement of the caring staff amazed me; it seemed as if they knew exactly what to do at what time and with whom, not allowing for any spare time to be wasted. They seemed to move like an orchestra, albeit without a conductor, or perhaps working ants constructing their anthill is a better analogy; every one of the caring staff knew their respective place in the totality of work that needed to be performed, without being told, and without having any doubts. At one point, there were nine caring staff workers in the hallway or in the large common room simultaneously, all delivering breakfast or medicine, making sure everything transpired as smoothly and effortlessly as possible. It seemed as if all nine caring staff members made sure the morning routine went according to plan, although there was no plan, at least not an explicit one. The sight of so many caring staff members working diligently and – not to be forgotten – in the «public» sphere of the unit, as opposed to being inside the respective residents´ rooms, was a stark contrast to the unit at any other time, later or earlier on that particular or any other day. In fact, only one hour later, at about 10.00, the hallway was, once again, deserted[13]. The caring staff had by then returned to the rooms of the residents, where they had spent most of their time up until 9.00, or were enjoying the first short coffee break of the day, in the large or small common room. Caring staff used the opportunity, the calm after the storm, to take a short break, but did not deem the situation as quite calm enough to take their break in the nurses´ station. In the large common room, they could spend five minutes talking to the residents who remained and were awake and alert, while two assisting nurses took advantage of the rare opportunity of the small common room being deserted by Maud, and sat down to read the paper.

Saturday, Acre Woods. My first whole Saturday spent at the nursing home. The day transpired differently compared to a normal weekday. There were five caring staff members present during the day-shift: one registered nurse, three assisting nurses and one assistant working on kitchen duty. The total level of staffing during the day-shift was slightly better than that of an evening-shift during a weekday and less than during day-shift on weekdays. During the evening-shift the five were replaced by two other assisting nurses and one assistant (it was said that one other assistant had called in sick, and was not replaced), which is one less caring staff member (including the absentee) than during evening-shift on a weekday. My general impression of the day was that it seemed like an endless evening-shift, both in atmosphere and the visibility of the staff in the «public sphere» of the unit. As a result of the relative low level of staffing compared to a normal day-shift, the caring staff had to suffice to attend to the most basic needs of the residents; making sure they were fed, visited the toilet and received their medication. The most noticeable part of the day, both during the day and evening, was the absence of the caring staff in the «public sphere» of the unit; they were hardly to be seen in the hallways or the common room. Rather, the caring staff members spent almost the entirety of their respective shifts in the rooms of residents, only seen outside when they were on their way to another resident's room or fetching food. The entirety of the respective shifts, with the exception of the latter half of the evening-shift, transpired as such. The caring staff did not seem to find time to spend in the common rooms or the hallway (and definitely not in the nurses' station), except for when bringing residents to and from the common rooms or the toilets.

---

13   Described elsewhere as «the great void» (translated from «det store tomrommet») (Hauge 2004), that is, the time after breakfast when caring staff leave the public sphere of the nursing home, leaving the remaining residents alone, to their dissatisfaction.

The few residents who did spent time in the common rooms, did so without the presence of caring staff for most of their time there. In addition to the absence of the caring staff, there were also noticeably fewer residents in the common rooms than during weekdays. Some of the residents walked to and from the common rooms on their own accord – influenced and perhaps somewhat unsettled by the lack of action and noise in the unit – while only two or three sat in the large common room for any length of time, as opposed to between four and eight, which was common during the weekdays.

The general atmosphere of the unit that Saturday, then, was markedly different from the weekdays; it was calm, quiet and uneventful. This general feeling was accentuated by the, for me, surprising lack of visitors on a Saturday, only two in total, which would be typical also for a weekday. It should also be noted that caring staff did not find time to have extensive breaks until about 17.00. In other words, caring staff working day-shift did not find time for lunch or any other breaks during the entire shift.

These examples illustrate how and why the everyday procedures, activities and schedules are experienced as hectic and strenuous for caring staff. Everyday life for caring staff *is* hectic and strenuous, both when considering the workload connected to a specific caring staff member's shift-plan (typically divided between day- and evening-shifts, sometimes, but seldom, including night-shifts), and when considering the total workload on the respective shifts including all caring staff. *But,* the respective shifts are hectic and strenuous in different ways; the weekday-shift is hectic and strenuous because of all the tasks and assignments placed there, *despite* the relative high level of staffing, while the weekend-shift is hectic and strenuous *because of* the low level of staffing. Despite both being considered hectic, the shifts are experienced as different both for caring staff and residents; the weekend-shift is even more hectic and strenuous than a day-shift during the weekday, as illustrated by the lack of breaks for the staff, the absence of staff presence in the «public sphere» and how residents are «kept» in their rooms.

More importantly still for our purposes is that the level of stress and bustle influences how residents are met and treated. The level of stress and bustle influences resident treatment for all shifts, though more visibly and explicitly when staffing levels are lower, as can be illustrated by the weekend-shift. During the weekend-shift the caring staff did not find time to prepare and bring the residents to the common rooms, especially residents who needed significant preparation and/or needed some form of supervision while being in the common room. In this sense, it was far more convenient for caring staff to have the residents with most needs in their rooms, where they could be controlled more easily. But it was also, in my opinion, necessary to keep them there; the few caring staff members could not keep an eye on the common room while tending to residents in their rooms; they were too few. Consequently, residents who did stay in the common rooms for shorter or longer periods of time, did so without the company of the caring staff, again, because they had to tend to residents with more pressing caring needs in their rooms. The caring staff were not in a position to solve this differently, in my opinion, given the level of staffing. The total caring needs of the residents were similar or equal to that of a weekday, while the level of staffing was significantly lower. Consequently, the caring staff had to attend to the most basic needs of the residents in their rooms.

Levels of staffing are, as seen from these examples, highly influential when considering not only the flow and development of everyday life at the nursing homes, including also, for lack of a better word, the atmosphere, but also how residents are met, treated and cared for by caring staff. Attending to the most basic needs of residents can be accomplished by relatively low levels of staffing, while attending to other needs, as seen in the difference between the two examples, implies higher levels of staffing. It is difficult to define what can be considered «low» and «high» levels of staffing, and what should be considered adequate staffing, as it is difficult to analyze todays nursing homes' levels of staffing in relation to caring needs of residents to yesterday's. However, *the effects of the relative difference of levels of staffing* at the same nursing home on different days and different shifts is both concrete and measurable. The relative difference in levels of staffing illustrates how levels of staffing to a significant degree determine what happens at a nursing home. When staffed at levels below those which caring staff consider adequate, and which we could say are in the best interest of the residents, nursing homes have to adopt routines and practices that are not ideal, for instance when it comes to when and how residents are «put to bed».

Acre Woods, approximately 15.30 on a weekday. There were four caring staff members present on the evening-shift, one registered nurse, two assisting nurses, and one student.

It was my impression that a vacant shift had not been filled because a student was present and considered an adequate substitute for the absentee (students were seldom part of the evening-shifts, but attended occasionally). It was a hectic evening, perhaps more so than usual, especially for the two assisting nurses. Meanwhile, the registered nurse was busy administering the medicine and tutoring the student. The registered nurse had earlier made an appointment with the student about going through the usual routines in the unit. She told an experienced assisting nurse that she and the student were on their way to the office of the unit leader. The assisting nurse replied: *But you have to wait a little bit, because I have to take Tanya to bed first,* implying that someone had to stay behind to watch over the large common room. Her tone of voice struck me as harsh, especially considering that the suggestion from the registered nurse seemed sensible, considering the relative calm in the unit at that particular time. Still, I was not completely surprised, knowing that the assisting nurse often spoke directly and freely. The registered nurse replied, not giving up without a fight: *But isn't that a bit early? We don't usually start until after 16.* The assisting nurse had already turned around walking towards the resident before the registered nurse had answered, and did not reply to her comment. The assisting nurse proceeded to accompany Tanya to bed, while the registered nurse and the student had to wait. Tanya, bound to her wheelchair with little mobility and speech, was the most anxious and easily unsettled of all the residents in the unit, and was almost always the first one to be accompanied to bed. Her calls and shouts from her room told us that the assisting nurse did not succeed in calming her in her room for well over an hour, while the assisting nurse went back and forth between Tanya's room and other residents in need of attention.

This specific example is not only illustrative of the negotiation between professional groups, perhaps taking the form of a contested rather than an internalized hierarchy but is also illustrative of the generating principles of routines in nursing homes. Caring staff adapt their routines and procedures because they have to, as they perceive it, based on the relatively low level of staffing. From the perspective of caring staff, then, routines and procedures are created based on staffing levels. From the perspective of residents, such routines and procedures are not individually adjusted, can be said to be too strictly implemented, and can thus be to the disadvantage of residents. As will be discussed, *routines* (and *rules*) can be seen as omnipresent in nursing homes, but also as adhering to different logic or ideology, thus producing confounding effects.

The general effects of levels of staffing on how residents are met and treated by caring staff are both systemic and specific. They are systemic in the sense of being routinized, illustrated by the predictability of the bed routines, especially for residents who do not have a say in the matter. They are specific and even mundane in the everyday incidents relating to how residents are greeted, talked to and helped. As such, caring staff adapt, explicitly and not, consciously or not, to the level of staffing in different ways, most notably by organizing the content of the shifts (primarily concerning the day-shifts), by adopting and executing a notion of primarily tending to the basic needs of residents, and by performing certain tasks based on suitability of the respective shift's schedule, rather than the interest of the respective residents.

A major challenge when it comes to such an organization, not yet discussed, is that one does not account for unforeseen events. As illustrated by Cate in Chapter 1, a day in the nursing home does not always transpire as planned; residents become ill or suddenly fall, which demands the attention of all or most of the caring staff present. There is, obviously, no way of planning for such events, but they will still occur, given the condition of residents. The state of balancing on the threshold of what can be considered attainable, is influenced and emphasized by the practice of not filling vacancies, again based on financial incentives. How the respective shifts can be said to balance on the threshold of attainability vary, then, not only based on intended levels of staffing (such as the difference between weekday-shift and weekend-shift), but also based on how many and which staff are present on the respective shifts. Furthermore, caring staff have to relate to whether or not the respective shifts will benefit from having temporary staff when vacancies occur. As such, the dilemma of filling vacancies or not, relates not only to financial incentives, but also to competence; having an unfamiliar temporary worker could imply an unwanted work burden for the experienced staff, measured against the potential benefit of having one extra staff member present.

The level of staffing, then, is not only about numbers. How the level of staffing affects residents is not only connected to the ratio between caring staff and residents. How residents are met and treated relates to an immensely important aspects touched on but not discussed in detail so far; the knowledge and experience of caring staff in relation to (the specific) residents, or *the continuity of care.*

The hardship and toil of the nursing home as experienced by caring staff is not simply discursive; it speaks to challenges with residents and challenges relating to staffing levels (which vary in time and place). A product of such challenges is the routinization of everyday life of nursing homes.

8.4. Meeting a resident: the anomaly of anomalies
Constance (see also the reading of the newspaper, Chapter 8.2)

Constance was an anomaly among the fellowship of residents, in several ways. Each resident is unique in their own way, has their own way of presenting themselves, has their own physical and cognitive ailments, and poses different challenges for caring staff. Still, Constance appeared to me as being particularly set off from the rest of the residents. Constance had a form of advanced dementia, making her disoriented, forgetful and restless. Her speech, however, was perfect, and her train of thought seemingly coherent and immediate, in contrast to many other residents. This gave her the appearance, at first glance, of being more present than she was, as her conversational partner would soon find out. Physically, there seemed to be nothing wrong with Constance; she was relatively young and walked on her own, having a comparatively good and straight posture, even when sitting. Among all the residents in the unit, Constance was the most mobile, both in capability and in action; she could and did move around constantly. The most peculiar aspect of Constance, compared to the other residents, was that it seemed that her dementia did not leave her confused, uneasy or nervous. Rather, it seemed to take a form of forgetfulness rather than confusion, a forgetfulness Constance either did not comprehend herself or simply chose not to allow to affect her. Constance was always in a good mood, despite being forgetful, disoriented and restless. She always looked for companions and was always smiling and cheerful. She gave the impression, explicitly and implicitly, of being content at the nursing home. Although such a way of presenting oneself might conceal both frustration and sadness, the difference between her and other residents, the latter often displaying feelings of discomfort and displeasure explicitly, remained noticeable.

The only thing missing from Constance's world, it would seem, were companions. She did not receive visitors, at least not on a regular basis, and found communicating with other residents difficult. It seemed to me that although Constance tried to connect with other residents constantly, she did not «match» them, as she was «too well-functioning» for the majority of residents who suffered from dementia and were lacking in language, and «not functioning enough» for the limited number of residents without dementia and language problems. When talking to the latter, as she often tried to do, she would quickly fall off the trail of the conversation, or lead it in a direction only understandable to herself, still smiling and seemingly content, to the dissatisfaction of her conversational partners. Because of Constance's derailments, they seldom took the initiative to talk to Constance. Constance's solitude among the residents led her to seek out staff members to talk with, relate to and connect with. Although seeing her explicit need for contact, staff seldom found time to talk to her for more than a few minutes at a time, often suggesting that she could go sit with other residents, or go to the large common room. Constance's shy demeanor probably contributed to the ease with which the staff would dismiss her, in addition to the busy schedule of the staff. Constance was, in my opinion, the resident who was the most affected by the busy schedule of the staff and their consequential lack of tending to the residents´ psychosocial needs, often sitting alone, alert and looking for someone to connect with.

Part three of the analysis: variation in practice

How things are done at the nursing home, relates to three overlapping levels of influence: *rules, routines* and *everyday practice.* These levels can be seen as co-dependent: rules form the premises of routines, which are formative for practice. Still, practice, the actual, everyday implementation of routines and rules, is the most significant in understanding *differences* between nursing homes. Practice, although internally shared, varies between nursing homes. Practice varies, in part, because it is strongly bounded by space; as will be illustrated through «the unit» and differences between units within a nursing home.

Variation in practice between nursing homes *can* occur; practice is by no means given by structural mechanisms or specific conditions, as seen in part two of the analysis. The overall structural framework of nursing homes; legislation and regulations, financial mechanisms as well as doxic representations of «the nursing home»; does not provide nursing homes with precise guidelines of action; they do not *determine* practice. The characteristics and composition of nursing home residents, as well as the varied and low level of staffing, provide an (intermediate) structural framework from which practice is created, *because it must*.

In this part, I will argue that variation is facilitated by the structure, resulting in a *fundamental uncertainty* for caring staff's implementation of practice. Such a fundamental uncertainty is met through the formation of *the institutional practice*; local and shared sets of practices for and by caring staff.

Continuity and stability, viewed as aspects of other discussed factors and conditions, influence the boundaries, formation, characteristics and strength of the institutional practice. Certain elements of continuity, particularly involvement of and with family and collaboration with physicians, can contribute to understanding and explaining variations of practices on hospitalization, while, at the same time, can be symptomatic of the more general institutional practice.

Practices of caring staff are generated (by necessity) by a *collective practical sense*, particularly actualized in nursing homes. Such a collective practical sense, which is seen as the generating principle of the institutional practice, can explain *differences* between nursing homes, also regarding hospitalizations.

The institutional practice

I will argue that nursing homes, and even units within a nursing home, *develop distinct, unique and internally shared sets of practices - the institutional practice.* The institutional practice is internally shared, although being implicit and unofficial.

The institutional practice is - in this book - both a premise and a result; both *that which will be explained* and *that which explains*. In this chapter, the formation and generating principles of the institutional practice will be outlined, explaining how and why it *is*, and how and why *it matters*. In Chapter 10, the institutional practice will be «used» to explain variations of practices, including that of hospitalization.

9.1. Rules and routines

But the institutional practice does not appear in a vacuum. Before the everyday practice in the nursing home, come the rules (the formal guidelines) and the routines (the quasi-official principles) organizing work. «Rules» will, in this context, include both legislation and regulations, and the specific and formalized procedures that nursing homes are obligated to implement and enforce from the respective municipalities. That means both the absolute principles which nursing homes and the agents operating within the boundaries of the nursing homes must adhere to (national legislation, for instance), and the more specific principles relating more directly to the organization of nursing homes. «Routines» will, in this context, be understood as the sets of written or unwritten principles guiding the everyday practice in nursing homes, as defined and implemented locally, by nursing homes or specific units. Routines can be similar to rules, as can their effect, but are distinct in the sense of not being created by explicit external demands. Routines are official, not always in the sense of being written, but by being shared and implemented by the practitioners; they are known by those who are responsible for their implementation.

9.1.1. Rules of conduct

The municipalities, although acting as the formal governing body, seldom interfere directly with the everyday operations of nursing homes. Our municipality has, for instance, suggested a maximum norm of staff per resident in nursing homes within the municipality. The specific institutions, however, can independently decide whether they want to follow this norm strictly (they will most likely not be sanctioned for deviating from the norm as long as they stay within their budget), and how they choose to interpret «staff per resident». As such, the institutions develop their own, independent systems of how many of the respective professional groups should be employed, on what shifts, and on what days, relating to but not mimicking the official regulation.

The specific institutions also create and maintain other rules, based on official guidelines but still adjusted locally. These include (though not exclusively): reporting schemes for residents (what should be documented for each resident at what time and where); workload for the staff (the structure of the shift plans, minimum coverage regulations for the respective professional groups); appearance of staff (use of uniforms, personalized items, and perfume, for instance); and visits by physicians (how and when, for private institutions). Depending on the size of the institution, the respective units may have some autonomy when it comes to these questions. Larger nursing homes usually leave it to the discretion of units when deciding how their days are organized, for instance when it comes to times for meals, report meetings, breaks for staff, delivering medication, and level and content of documentation. In sum, the organization of everyday life in nursing homes is shaped by the demands of external and internal rules, connected to a wider trend of bureaucratization within the public healthcare sector, to which nursing homes relate differently (see also Slagsvold 1986). However, although inexplicably shaped by rules, the respective institutions have a significant degree of discretion in their adjustment and implementation of rules.

Many of the rules to which nursing homes must relate can be seen by practitioners as inadequate. They can be inadequate both with regard to content (degree of detail, for instance) and function (who they serve and benefit). Nursing homes as institutions, though serving as an agent of the resident, must also safeguard other interests, which in some instances might be contradictory to the best interests of residents (Freiman & Murtaugh 1993, see also Kayser-Jones 1990). Similarly, the rules pertaining to the organization and operation of nursing homes can be experienced as being in a competitive relationship with or even contradictory to the main objectives of the caring staff. Rules addressing shift plans, minimum staffing ratios for respective professional groups, the use of replacement staff and the ordering of goods (food and equipment), for instance, can be construed as having the inherent function of being cost-effective for the institution rather than primarily being in place for the betterment of residents, although being generally presented as implemented for purposes of «quality improvement» (Jacobsen 2005, Vike 2003). The ordering of food will serve as an example of what is considered a general dynamic.

Many nursing homes in our municipality have outsourced the preparation of warm meals for their residents; the meals were previously made in a large kitchen serving the entire nursing home. This new arrangement is thought to be more cost-effective, and, ideally, should free up time for caring staff to spend on residents (or alternatively, wages can be moved from kitchen staff to caring staff). Most of our nursing homes had implemented this new regime; only one out of six, Acre Woods, still prepared dinner on site. These nursing homes now must order meals from a larger nursing home not included in the sample. Twice a week caring staff in the units, more often than not assisting nurses, have to spend hours ordering meals for each resident respectively, detailing personal preferences for each meal, through electronic forms, as opposed to being served warmed meals from an on-site kitchen. This is done during the caring staff's allocated time with residents in the units; assisting nurses do not get extra time, or extra manpower, to perform these tasks, but have to find time in between other responsibilities. Consequently, assisting nurses will choose not to perform certain tasks that are not on the absolute top of the «to-do-list», more often than not spending time with residents in the common areas between meals. Meanwhile, the act of ordering food, as opposed to the «breaks» with residents, is not a responsibility that can be dropped or even postponed:

Late morning, approximately 9.30-11.30, at Galactic Manor. Breakfast is finished, all residents have moved or been moved from the kitchen area. Of the ten residents in the unit, eight attended breakfast in the kitchen area, while two were served in their rooms, as they are bedridden. Four of the eight residents have retired to their rooms, while the other four have moved (two by their own accord, two with help from staff) to the adjacent common area, a spacious and nicely decorated large room with two sofa groups and a large television, which serves as the centerpiece of the room.

Two of the residents sit quietly on a sofa, nodding off, while two sit in front of the television: one in a wheelchair, one in a regular chair placed there by staff. They appear to be paying attention to the television, showing local news from the public broadcaster, NRK. None of the four residents interact with each other, nor do they pay attention to my presence.

In the kitchen area, partly visible from the common room (staff can pay attention to the common room from the kitchen area from one part of the kitchen, and can hear most of what goes on there) one solitary staff member, a female assisting nurse, is sitting by the large dining table. She is taking notes on a form while going to and from the kitchen cabinets and appears to be cross-referencing with another list she has. She acknowledges me and says that *it's time to order again.* She is alone; no other staff member is visible nor can they be heard in the kitchen, the common room or the hallways. Even though I know the answer, I ask *where are the others?* She replies that they are busy attending to patients in their rooms. I sit down at the end of the large table, giving her space to work while still letting it be known that I am interested in what is going on. For about two hours, she continues with her work, filling out her form while checking her list and the kitchen cabinets. Meanwhile, she talks about what she is doing and makes short comments on her thoughts about the tasks. *We have to do this twice a week. It's a lot of work because there are so many details. A lot of the patients need special food, or they do not like or want this and that. So there are a lot of details.* She tells me that it is usually her job, if she is on day-shift, if not, somebody else has to do it *and that can be a hassle because it's easy to mess it up.* When asked why she is the one responsible, she responds: *I'm not sure. It kind of just started out with me doing it, and then went from there. Now I just do it, I guess.* While she does the job, lasting at least two hours, the unit is remarkably quiet. The residents in the common area remain there, hardly making any sound. No other residents are visible nor can be heard, and staff are hardly to be seen. A couple of nurses pass by quickly, fetching whatever they need for their assignments or delivering short messages to the assisting nurse. After over one hour of continuous documentation, I comment that *it seems like a lot of work…* She smiles, lets out a little laugh and responds: *Yes. It is. But what can you do?* After a while, I ask: *But it's so quiet here, isn't it? What if it wasn't, what if you had to help with the patients all this time?* She shrugs: *Honestly, well it´s not easy. If I have to help, I'll help of course, but it doesn't add up, you know.* Only at the end of this period, at about 11.15, staff and a couple of residents, accompanied by staff, start to fill the kitchen and common areas, preparing for lunch. Meanwhile, the four residents have been sitting quietly sleeping, dozing off or watching television, not making any calls or other attempts to contact the staff.

The outsourcing of food, defined as within the domain of «rules» by being an obligatory (for public institutions) or voluntary (for private institutions) part of a larger municipal scheme, can, as such, produce effects which are contrary to the priorities of caring staff, and, perhaps, the best interests of residents. Based on the example, and by sentiments voiced by themselves (at the included and other nursing homes), caring staff must spend more time on administration and less time on residents because of this arrangement. While the argument that such arrangements leading to less time spent on residents than before can be debated (especially concerning difficulties in measuring such effects), the sentiments caring staff remains clear and strong; they would prefer, for their own and the residents' sake, not to have them.

Other rules and regulations, especially concerning the multi-faceted documentation procedures concerning residents, can be construed as having the inherent function of «protecting» the institution from potential criticism, whether from family or media (Lloyd et al. 2014), and not primarily, at least not solely, being for the benefit of staff or residents. The specific effects of the implementation of rules, consequently, are not necessarily seen as beneficial for staff or for residents: the strict and detailed procedures for documentation of residents can, as for the outsourcing of food, limit time available for direct staff-to-resident interaction. At such, rules can produce unintended consequences, sometimes in direct opposition to the primary objectives of caring staff.

9.1.2. The routines of everyday life

For residents and staff in nursing homes the everyday flow (who does what, at what time and with whom) is remarkably similar from day to day, as seen in the presentation of a typical day. Elsewhere, it has been demonstrated that caring staff are bound to their daily routines, always knowing what to do in a mutual and automated sense (Sandvoll 2013: 16-18). Although the work shifts vary on a daily or weekly basis for most staff, the days at the nursing home are hard to tell apart. Weekends differ somewhat, not so much when it comes to the everyday flow of activities, but rather when it comes to number of staff (fewer), visitors (more, although only at some nursing homes) and organized leisure activities (fewer). The repetitiveness of daily life might be interpreted as boring and mundane from the point of view of the outsider, but it also gives the caring staff predictability, and allows them to cope with what they voice as an uneven distribution of workload and number of staff. For the residents, repetitiveness of daily life can also be a comfort.

> Emerald Gardens, in the common area/dining area at 9.30 in the morning. Breakfast is finished for most residents, although a majority still sit at the table, finishing their coffee or talking to the caring staff, two of whom are still present. Meanwhile, the other staff members are in the rooms of bedridden residents. The activity worker has just entered, and is preparing for the daily activity of reading the newspaper and subsequent quiz. An elderly resident enters, a well-groomed «gentleman», particularly popular with both the female residents and the caring staff. He joyfully greets everyone, wishing a *Good morning on this beautiful day.* He sits down at his regular place (one of four free places at the table), and continues to take center stage, something he appears to be well accustomed to, by asking loudly: *Well, well, well, what's for breakfast today? Eggs, I hope.* One of the caring staff replies that he can have eggs if he wants, and prepares one for him. An assistant sitting close to me (by a smaller table some distance from the larger dining table) approaches me, while smiling and seemingly amused by the situation: *You know he just had a full breakfast twenty minutes ago.*

Predictability and repetitiveness can be a comfort to residents; perhaps they are used to that from their former life, or perhaps it comforts residents with dementia in a constant battle to make sense of their surroundings. Similarly, predictability and repetitiveness can be a comfort for staff, trying to deal with the challenges connected to «the toil» of the nursing home.

Irrespective of whether the repetitiveness of daily life is viewed as positive or negative for residents and staff, it is still prevalent; everyday life in nursing homes is organized and structured by activities, actions and tasks that take place at the same time, every day, regardless of who performs them. In this sense, *time* is the principle by which nursing homes are organized, while other factors, most notably *who* the participants are, are secondary. This principle relates primarily to the *organization* of everyday life, while the *form of the actual practice* – what, as opposed to how it goes on – to a far greater extent relates to *who the participants are.*

The repetitiveness of nursing home life is influenced by more than formal and concrete guidelines and recommendations, as represented by *the rules.* More than anything else, the repetitiveness relates to a wide range, but also coherent, sets of informal and self-governed (by the institution or the unit) *routines*, as visible in the excerpt of a typical day in the unit. Caring staff know what to do, when to do it, and whom to do it to, without the help of written guidelines. Through the implementation of routines, the ebb and flow of daily life in nursing homes repeats itself. One day follows the next, with little separating them, except perhaps for the persons wearing the uniforms. For the residents, nursing home life is monotonous, mundane and repetitive, for better or worse. The routines of nursing home life are omnipresent, often taken for granted by those who perform them, perhaps with the exception of the neophyte; but she also embraces the routines, in an attempt to integrate herself into the environment. Routines, then, are the guiding principle of work, a principle according to which work is measured. For staff, routines are measures from which one should not deviate, perhaps as opposed to rules. For the caring staff in nursing homes, the routines are *what we do*; they are theirs. Routines differ from the more formal rules, not necessarily by how agents relate actively to them, but rather in how agents experience a sense of belonging and closeness to them. As such, routines are not problematized (Harnett et al. 2012: 44) as rules might be, and they are actively used, whereas rules might not be.

But not everything the staff do in nursing homes is part of their routines; not all actions are routinized. There is, I will argue, an aspect of everyday performance that is more subtle, more implicit and less instrumental. While the boundaries between them are indistinct and changing, a division between routines and *an institutional practice*, to be outlined in Chapter 9.5, can be drawn. In short, routines are the organizational framework guiding the everyday actions of caring staff, while an institutional practice will be understood as *how agents act*, given, among other factors, the routines they relate to. As such, *practice* can be understood as the actual implementation of routines. Practice, in my understanding, is inherently unreflective, while routines entail a higher degree of reflection. This distinction is subtle, but important; practice entails more than the adherence to habitual patterns.

9.2. Locality and boundaries of routines and practice

The agents, regardless of conscious deliberation, are gradually accustomed to the routines of daily life, and, from the perspective of the outsider, seem to welcome it. But whose routines are they? To what extent are routines shared in a specific nursing home, or even a unit? To what extent are routines shared among (similar) nursing homes? To what extent are routines as an abstract, theoretical phenomenon, shared and used among nursing homes, while the specific content of the routines might differ? These are important questions, as the locality and boundaries of routines can contribute to uncovering from where and how the more subtle and immeasurable everyday practice is generated. For instance: the specific incidents of hospitalization of nursing home residents can be seen either as adhering to the routines of daily life, or, in cases of meeting the unknown or unexpected, as ways in which the taken for grantedness of routines suddenly becomes a matter of active deliberation. This might be when a «new» or complicated situation arises or when inexperienced staff must relate to making quick decisions. In these exceptional cases, the routines of the institution are insufficient. In these instances, creating a space for a discussion of that which is not discussed, a local, shared and implicit institutional practice becomes explicit.

Everyday life in nursing homes is repetitive, routinized and mundane; the staff know what to do next, and residents, if in possession of the cognitive capacity to do so, know what to expect next. That is not to say that actions are not discussed or planned for, but rather that the internal framework of the staff's practice, who does what and at what general time, is shared among the staff and implemented by the staff without much active deliberation. It is more or less taken for granted. As seen from the excerpt of daily life at a nursing home, staff have to plan certain aspects of their day, especially related to specific delegation of tasks, while *how* things are done is left unspoken. However, how things are done *is not unknown* to those about to act. This *knowing without being explicitly taught,* leaves us with somewhat of a puzzle: from where does the practice come? Given that practice is shared, what are the boundaries of that which is shared?

9.2.1. The units

To analyze the boundaries of routines and practice, different units within the same nursing home can be a practical starting point. That being said, the organization of units, including the division between them, differs greatly between nursing homes, as within our small sample. Some nursing homes, primarily the larger ones, have units operating more or less independently from others; caring staff do not rotate between units, and do not, generally, concern themselves with the operation of the nursing home outside the boundaries of the unit. Smaller nursing homes might rotate staff between units more frequently, or even not have staff assigned to units at all; they work where needed on any given day. It is also typical in smaller nursing homes for all staff to have greater knowledge of what goes on in other units, whether it is related to residents, staff or the organization of work. Norwegian nursing homes (and keep in mind that Norwegian nursing homes on average are quite small, relatively speaking) are often somewhere between the extremes; they are typically divided into distinguishable units, while residents, unit leaders, and most of the caring staff are designated to their respective units. Caring staff usually have some form of formal flexibility (being employed at the nursing home rather than the unit, for instance), or informal flexibility (being employed in the unit, but still overlapping when needed, for instance) regarding where they «belong», thus securing some degree of overlap in knowledge and experience between units.

The organization and independence of units do not, however, only depend on nursing home size, but also on the physical space of the nursing homes. Units might be placed on different floors, or be far from each other on the same floor, not easily accessible, especially for residents. Other nursing homes have a more «open» layout; units are close to each other and connected through an open, easily accessible common area, with little delineating the boundaries of one unit from the next. Regardless of whether the physical layout of the nursing home provides clear boundaries between units, the units are usually given their distinct identity not only in name, but also in decoration, most notably different color schemes for each unit. Furthermore, the overall physical layout of nursing homes is obviously connected to when they were built, and whether they were built as a nursing home, or later refurbished as one. The physical layout of nursing homes can often be traced back to the architectural trends in the period when they were built, in other words. The autonomy of the unit, then, is connected to size and to the physical layout of the nursing home, but these do not necessarily overlap: small nursing homes can have units with relative autonomy *and* have units without clear boundaries between them, depending on the overall physical layout of the nursing home. However, the same does not necessarily hold true for large nursing homes, where units tend to be clearly separated from each other. Some of our nursing homes can serve as examples:

1: Cloud House:

Cloud House can serve as an example of an ill-fitted architectural design for a nursing home. It was originally built as an apartment complex, and was recently refurbished as a nursing home, while maintaining most of the interior walls. Consequently, the hallways are far too narrow, not allowing, for example, for caring staff to support a resident on each side while walking down the hallway, a support several of the residents need. Furthermore, the units are separated clearly from each other, by floor and by a hallway not easily navigable for residents or staff. Likewise, the elevator, one of the most important features for all nursing homes, is not placed so as to directly enter the units from it. Residents are therefore not mobile, while staff have to spend a lot of time going from one place to the next during the day. Consequently, staff generally stay in their respective units. There are no easily accessible areas, common rooms for instance, where residents and staff can meet across units. There is a large common area in an adjacent part of the building, but this is difficult to access, partly because of the ineffective placement and size of the elevator, and is rarely used.

2: Emerald Gardens:

The building itself is very old, and actually consists of several small buildings and add-ons, not visible before entering. The main building was not built as a nursing home, but rather a large villa. Combined, this makes for a very eclectic and varied physical layout inside the nursing home, far from the «clean» architectural designs of modern nursing homes. However, because of the way it has been refurbished, residents, staff and family members all state that it is functional and to their liking. There is a lot of open space so that residents can walk freely and easily from their rooms to the large common area, and even to other units. Staff can move quickly from their designated unit to the common area, other units, and the nurses work station. The common area also allows for a good overview of the nursing home as a whole. Perhaps as a consequence of this physical layout, the caring staff often contribute to other units than the one they are assigned to. Staff can easily access other units, and some of the more mobile residents are also, at times, in other units, a rare sight in most other nursing homes.

3: Galactic Manor:

As opposed to the previous two examples, this nursing home building is new and was originally built as a nursing home. The architectural layout and the general aesthetics of the interior, therefore, are different from the two previous examples: it is neat, color coordinated, functional, and common rooms are for the most part easily accessible. When entering, the visitor immediately gets the impression of being in an «institution». One peculiar aspect of the layout, however, stands out. There are three units in the nursing home, two on one floor and one on another, the latter of which also houses the administration. The two units on the same floor are connected by hallways without doors separating them, making moving between them easy for staff and residents alike. Aside from those familiar with the nursing home, one would not get the impression of there being two separate units on the floor. Consequently, staff in the units, although formally employed in the specific units, often help in the adjacent unit; ask for help and advice, and interact socially with staff from the other unit. Residents, however, do not interact much across units, but are familiar with the staff from the adjacent unit. The third unit, on the other hand, is more secluded. It is, as mentioned, on another floor, and there is little if no mobility between the floors, at least not to the same extent as between the two other units. As opposed to the first nursing home, but similar to the second, there are no large common areas for residents outside of the units. However, as opposed to the second nursing home, the common areas inside the units are spacious and often used.

4: Acre Woods:

The building is old, but has seen extensive periods of refurbishment and redecorating since it was built, and now has the interior look of a modern institution. Being significantly larger than the aforementioned institutions, the building itself and the interior create a first impression of being an «institution», in accordance with the notion previously discussed. The units are clearly separated from each other by floor, by locked doors at the points of entry, by large nameplates at the points of entry, and by different color schemes on each floor. Other units are not easily accessible as they are separated by a hallway, always locked, and not part of the units themselves. The staff can move between floors by an elevator, directly accessible through the corridors in the units, but these are off-limits to the residents, leaving staff with some level of mobility, residents with little. Given this physical layout and the size of the nursing home, units are clearly separated; staff are employed in the respective units and do not interact much with staff from other units, either to help with different tasks or socially. In addition, because of the size of the nursing home, there are two physicians employed, each responsible for their respective units, further contributing to the absence of the mobility of knowledge and experience between units (for the other three nursing homes mentioned, there is only one physician employed). Unit leaders do attend administrative meetings together, but they do not generally concern themselves with the day-to-day operation of the units.

These examples highlight the differences in physical layout and architectural design between nursing homes, and how units are organized accordingly. Although they are not randomly selected, more nursing homes could be added, which would add to the variation in physical layout and organization of units: *a nursing home is not a nursing home*. More to the point: nursing homes do not only vary in looks and buildings, they also vary, significantly, in how units – the actual home of the residents – are organized and function. Units come in different sizes, forms and colors (literally), but also function differently in regard to how they relate to other units and/or to the entirety of respective nursing homes.

9.2.2. The unit as a community of staff or community of units?

The significance of units in nursing homes cannot, however, be reduced to physicality; the unit is more than its appearance and the division of units is about more than the walls between them. The unit is, to varying degrees, a community (primarily) of caring staff.

As discussed, caring staff can experience alienation from the process of defining the premises of their place of work, resulting at times in opposition or even apathy. But being alienated can also have the opposite effect; it can produce strategies of ingenuity and originality, grounded in the need for defining a sense of collective identity, a sense of commonness. Such a need, the pragmatic effect of which is the coping mechanism of routines described in the previous chapter, can also result in communal sentiments among caring staff, described elsewhere as «*the fellowship of poverty*» among staff in nursing homes (Jacobsen 2005).

Lindgren's description of «*the clinic*»[1] (1992) can assist us in conceptualizing how such affinities are structured. At «*the clinic*», having a defined hierarchy between segregated professional groups, the lowest in the hierarchy

---

[1] «*The clinic*» refers to a hospital, constructed by the author, highlighting similarities between several hospitals included in the study (Lindgren 1992).

(equivalent to our assistants and assisting nurses) develop a sense of unity based on a *«culture of collectivity»*: a collective where similarity and equality bind members, not necessarily in explicit opposition to others higher in the hierarchy, but still in relation to them. The culture of collectivity develops from powerlessness through the creation of unity and togetherness among those not in a position of power. The culture of collectivity is not ambitious (in the sense of seeking positional change connected to other professional groups in the hierarchy), a trait separating the collective culture from *«the cooperative culture»* - the middle level of the hierarchy (equivalent to our registered nurses). The cooperative culture is, to a higher degree, based on vertical affinity both internally and externally. Members within the culture are ascribed different statuses, as opposed to the equality of the collective culture, while, at the same time, the culture is unified by having a common aim; the relative position of the group in relationship to others.

Lindgren's description of the respective cultures and the system of cultures is illustrative and, to some degree, transferable to the systems of integration and segregation within and between professional groups at our nursing homes. In my opinion, we can identify collective and cooperative cultures in our nursing homes, although in different ways than for «the clinic»[2]. *The relationship* between the two cultures *varies* within our sample of nursing homes, pointing to an important difference in how community and affinity are created and played out within small and large nursing homes, respectively.

In smaller nursing homes affinity is bound to the institution. Individual and group identity is directed towards the institution as a whole rather than the units, in contrast to larger nursing homes. The community – the nursing home – is, like «the clinic», simultaneously integrated and segregated. It serves as an entity to which the respective members belong, but is simultaneously divided into professional groups (with specific tasks ascribed to them) *integrated on the level of the institution*, thus creating differences towards other professional groups also integrated on the level of the institution. As such, smaller nursing homes tend to have elements both of the collective and the cooperative culture, somewhat different from «the clinic». The collective culture refers to an affinity towards

---

2   It should also be noted that the three levels of hierarchy within «the clinic»: «flickor», «systrar» and «doctorer» (physicians), do not fit, formally, with my definition of «caring staff» (consisting of assistants, assisting nurses and registered nurses, leaving out physicians), but are still translated as such, since physicians have a smaller part (in numbers and influence) in nursing homes than in hospitals.

the institution, while the cooperative cultures can be found within each respective professional group (and not simply the middle group). At larger nursing homes, where one would assume that professional groups to a larger degree are separated and internally integrated, a different dynamic is at play; for nursing homes of a certain size, the entity of community and affinity is the unit, rather than the nursing home. Affinity across professional groups is strengthened within the unit, while «the others» is constructed as being other units or management, rather than other professional groups. A culture of collectivity and a culture of cooperative, therefore, are, integrated *into* the community of the unit, while the nursing home in its entirety can be described as a loosely integrated culture of cooperativeness, although not to the extent present in «the clinic».

Depending on the nursing home, then, boundaries of collective identities *can be more or less isolated to units*. The *need* to define a collective identity, which relates to the process of inclusion and exclusion, can be related to the unit rather than the nursing home as a whole. The unit can, in some nursing homes, become the primary entity of identification for caring staff; the unit is where caring staff work, but it can also be the place where they feel connected, where their loyalty lies, and to where they «belong». Thus, caring staff in some nursing homes will spontaneously refer to their unit when describing «us», also sometimes, in smaller nursing homes.

9.2.3. Practice in the unit

The process of collective identification is not only strongly connected to *who we are*, but also, perhaps more than anything else, to *what we do*: to practice. Work for caring staff is filled with minor and major tasks that are performed in certain ways, as opposed to other, possible ways. *Who we are*, therefore, is strongly connected to *what we do*. In the eyes of the caring staff, then, the collective identity is defined by shared ways of performing everyday tasks and activities. Furthermore, *the collective* point of referral when describing practice, referring to *us* rather than individual practices, is of significance. Practice in the unit is almost without exception described as a *collective endeavor*, making the central collective entity for caring staff «the unit», and, *simultaneously*, making the unit a fellowship.

The unit, then, is the main entity from which collective identity is defined, the degree of which will vary, depending on the organization of units at the respective nursing homes (which again depends on the size and physical layout of the nursing home). Units *can* differ within the same nursing home. Units can differ within the same nursing home, even though they have the same resources and are equal in all other formal aspects.

To further emphasize how collective identities and a sense of community are found on the unit level, by creating informal distinctions and barriers to other units, the example can be used of a nursing home where the *formal* division of units is not very distinct, Galactic Manor. As mentioned, two of the units are on the same floor, with no barriers separating them and some mobility of staff between them. The units have the same physical layout, the same decoration, the same colors, and the same level of staffing. In appearance, the units are mirror images of each other. Even so, the units are different. A note from doing fieldwork at both units:

> It is noticeable how different the two units are. I walk a lot between them during day and evening shifts, which is easy and quickly done, making the differences between them all the more apparent. An assistant nurse told me, somewhat jokingly, that their unit is much more *structured*, and that things are more organized there. I share her opinion. They have a strict schedule of how they organize the day, which is much more dependent on what time it is, while the other unit lets the residents control the tempo and flow of the day to a much higher degree. Or perhaps I am interpreting too much; perhaps the other unit is just less structured? Having different residents with regard to functional ability would perhaps explain the difference, but management is supposed to distribute residents evenly between units. I believe that the residents, rather, are perceived as different not because of their different functional abilities, but because of how they are treated and cared for. In the «unstructured unit», residents are more active, talking, watching television and interacting with the staff. Residents in the «structured unit» are more sedated, they tend to doze off in the common room without anyone to talk to, while the staff spend more time in the kitchen area. Residents seem to be less stimulated by the staff, who have a hard time finding enough time for resident interaction. But there is also something else at play; it is not just about the level of «structure», the units «feel» different. Even though they are closely connected and similar, there is a different atmosphere from one to the next. It is difficult to explain, but still quite apparent; the atmosphere is distinctly different, one more relaxed and serene, the other busier and more formal.

Units are, like nursing homes, different, adhering differently to structural frameworks and institutional conditions, having different organizational modes, different levels of staffing and, perhaps, different resident demographics. But units within the same nursing homes are generally very similar, at least at first glance. They are usually designed to be mirror images of each other with nothing else dividing them apart from different colors on the walls. Units within the same nursing home are usually built alike; having the same architectural layout, including similar number and size of resident and common rooms. They are usually staffed alike; having the same number of total staff and a similar composition of staff (from the respective professional groups). They also «recruit» residents from the same local area through the same local governing office, often evenly divided between units based on the respective nursing homes' interpretation of the total level of caring needs in their respective units. Formally, then, units are similar, in all apparent aspects. Still, units develop distinct and different attributes, connected both to different and differing «spirits of the place» and different ways of relating to their residents.

To understand how such differences develop and are implemented, we must understand how units relate to *other units*, to the nursing home and to the doxic notion of «the nursing home». The primary unit, called *the unit*, where a majority of the fieldwork was spent (approximately four months), will serve as an example of how a unit includes and excludes, and, consequently, how communities are developed in relation to other units and the institution in its entirety. Before discussing the particularity of *the unit*, a brief presentation of its characteristics will be given (for reasons of anonymity, certain minor and major aspects of these have been left out, while some minor aspects have been altered).

The unit is one of several at Acre Woods. It is, like the other units in the nursing home, relatively large, in physical size and number of residents. It does not, as most other nursing homes, adhere to the official norm of having small units of 8-12 residents (see Chapter 3). *The unit* is separated from other units and other parts of the nursing home by floors, accessible through a stairwell and an elevator. Still, it is relatively easy for staff to move around to other units, to the administration and to the activity center, as both the stairwell and the elevator are easily accessible. There are three common rooms in the unit, one large and two small. The large common room is used for all the meals, activities and other social gatherings. It is also commonly used by some of the residents in between mealtimes, although it is not always clear whether or not it is at their own, or the staff's, behest. One of the smaller common rooms is placed centrally in the unit and is inhabited by a small group of residents from early morning to late afternoon, almost every day. The last common room is placed at the end of the hallway, and usually only used at mealtimes. At the center of the unit lies a long, straight and wide corridor, with resident rooms on each side. At the center of this corridor is the large common room, one of the small common rooms, the elevator, the nurses' station and the office of the unit leader, all in relatively short distance from each other.

The residents have, as mentioned earlier, their own and independent rhythms of everyday life, from which they rarely deviate. They usually sit at the same places, at the same time, with the same co-residents, regardless of whether it is mealtime or not[3]. Thus, the movement of the unit, who does what, where and at what time, is fairly predictable. The different rooms are usually also inhabited by the same small «groups» of residents, especially one of the small and, to some degree, the large common room. The small common room has a particular stable group of residents, a group of cognitively clear and well-functioning residents, making it, together with the positioning of the room, a centerpiece of social activity in the unit. The large common room is usually inhabited by several residents, but «membership» shifts more compared to the small common room. As opposed to the smaller common room, residents in the large one are often placed there at the staff's desire, rather than because of their own desire. In general the residents are, as in other units and other nursing homes, a mixed group when it comes to level of physical and cognitive ability. Everyone, however, has some sort of physical or cognitive impairment (the severity of which varies) if not, they simply would not be there. The residents themselves draw a clear line between residents who are «clear and present», and those who are not. For the residents, at least those who are «clear and present», there is no in-between, you are either defined within their group or not, and there is no return once you have left (see also Bjelland 1982). Those who consider themselves «clear and present», all have some sort of physical impairment, while the opposite is not necessarily true.

The staff working specifically in *the unit* is a mixed group of registered nurses, assisting nurses and assistants. There is a wide gap in level of experience within and between these groups, but in general, turnover in the unit is low, especially for registered

---

3 The predictability of seating arrangements for residents at mealtimes has been described elsewhere as resembling that of the parking lot at a place of work: workers park in their designated places, automatically and without deliberation (Hauge 2004).

nurses and assisting nurses. The large majority of staff are women, born in Norway and living in the municipality. There is a growing number of female assisting nurses and assistants in the unit born in other countries, mostly from Africa and Southeast Asia, a trend that the nursing home shares with other nursing homes in the municipality. There are a few male assistants and one assisting nurse (born abroad), but only the latter has a full-time position. In general, though, most staff have permanent positions, although many only work part-time. In addition to the staff working specifically in the unit, staff working at the nursing home in general are often visible during shorter or longer parts of the day, primarily during the day-shift. A physician visits the unit one day a week and is available most other days. Cleaning staff work in the units during different intervals of the day. Maintenance staff work in the unit at more irregular intervals, depending on what needs to be done. A priest visits about once a month (but is also regularly in the activity center). Activity personnel visit the unit once a week and entertain the residents for a couple of hours.

This brief description of some of the most notable features of *the unit* can be read together with the excerpt of a day in *the unit*, presented in Chapter 3. While giving a descriptive introduction to the features and activities in *the unit*, these do not reveal what distinguishes it from other units. The differences between units can be approached through the perspectives of caring staff: for the caring staff, the entity from which identity is ascribed is *their unit*, and what defines their unit stands in relation to *other units at the nursing home*. When describing their unit, for instance, caring staff will implicitly and explicitly compare their unit to other units at the nursing home and highlight aspects that set their unit apart from the rest. In this particular unit, one defining characteristic is dominant over all others; how staff in the unit relate to dying residents. In the eyes of leadership of *the unit,* this position is strongly connected to the physician and how he relates to the topic:

An interview with the assisting unit leader of *the unit*. Interviews, primarily with top- and middle management, were carried out both at the start and at the end of data collection, before and after fieldwork, that is (see Chapter 1). This particular interview, meanwhile, took place after more than four months of fieldwork in the particular unit. The interviewee, therefore, knew of me and my project, leading to difficulties in getting beyond that which is taken for granted between the interviewer and the interviewee, while also leading to opportunities to get past, to a certain extent, official accounts. The assisting unit leader is a person of action rather than words; to the point, somber and «professional» when talking to me and to colleagues, often giving short matter-of-fact answers. One topic during our conversation did spur an interest in her, however, producing an uncommonly detailed and opinionated reply. Earlier in the conversation, we had talked about how her unit organizes everyday activities. She had raised the subject of another unit, to exemplify how they organized differently. I then proceeded to ask her if there *is more to it than organization?*

The assisting unit leader: *We in the unit have a different attitude than the other units. It has a lot to do with the physicians, but also with leaders. We two leaders are much aligned and agree that we do not have to treat at all cost. We can do this because the physician agrees with us. He is easy to relate to, and is on the same wavelength as us. In the other unit[4] they hospitalize faster and use much more intravenous therapy and an aggressive approach. The physician there is more positive towards hospitalizations, while we think that it is not always the best choice. And sometimes we have seen that the hospitals agree with us, because they come back almost immediately.*

While the assisting unit leader highlighted the role of the physician in how *the unit* is positioned towards treatment, other caring staff in *the unit*, not in positions of leadership (and thereby not cooperating directly with the physician), highlight a consensus between caring staff as central for *the unit's* positioning towards treatment. For the assisting unit leader, what defines their unit is connected to what they do; to their practice. The defining characteristics are not based on the appearance of *the unit*, nor by its inhabitants, staff or residents. The defining characteristics are not based on *how* it is to be in *the unit*, its feeling or its atmosphere, nor by its rules and formal characteristics. For the staff, it is based on *what they do*, every day. And what they do – their practice – is understood *in relation to what others do*, others that are close by; other units at the nursing home.

To caring staff in *the unit*, what they do and how they do it, is an alternative to other ways of doing, and is therefore significant in defining the identity of *the unit*, as seen in relation to other units. What is being done in *the unit* is, in this sense, a communal activity; it is shared by its participants (inside *the unit*), and not by others (outside *the unit*). The insider, then, understands and presents collective identity as being generated on the level of the unit. The unit is understood and presented in relation to other units at the nursing home, in

---

4   Refers to a neighboring unit discussed previously in the conversation.

contrast to the emic approach of the visitor; highlighting its relational rather than its inherent features.

Specifically, what the assisting unit leader points to as a defining characteristic – an approach of less medical treatment of severely ill or dying residents – not only points to this; the shared practice in *the unit*, but also to a positioning concerning the general dilemma of care versus medicalization, discussed earlier. The dilemma of care versus medicalization again relates to the potentialities of specific treatment regimens for residents. The treatment of the nursing home resident, or, as is the case in many situations; *whether or not to treat the nursing home resident*, is a complex matter, further complicated by the absence of protocols and directives guiding the agent.

9.3. Practice and uncertainty

Practice in nursing homes has a strong local component, through sentiments of community and collectivity shared at the nursing home or in the unit. However, *the dynamics of the formation of practices*, has not been discussed. Why are patterns of practice developed and implemented locally, as opposed to being generic patterns of actions, shared at larger nursing homes or even between nursing homes? For they, units and nursing homes, are essentially similar entities and institutions: having similar function and meaning attached to them, adhering to the same structural framework (rules or the educational system), and being viewed and presented similarly by the outsider.

9.3.1. Practice in uncertainty

The practices of caring staff are not given. There are few ready-made solutions. Many of the actions and decisions during a day, especially concerning the deteriorating health of a resident are filled with *uncertainty*. Such an uncertainty arises from a primary sense of detachment from the general *and* specific structural frameworks at play in nursing homes. Caring staff in nursing homes must relate to rules and regulations (primarily the national health legislation and municipal regulations), guidelines and expectations from «above» and outside. These might be specific (in the form of specific regulations) or more conceptual (in the form of official discourses and popular notions about «the nursing home»). Combined they create a framework from which nursing homes are shaped, and to which caring staff must relate. But caring staff are not involved in creating, transferring or adapting these specific and conceptual notions to the nursing home. Even minor aspects of everyday life in nursing homes, such as the organization of ordering goods as discussed, are not made by practitioners in need of the goods, but rather by management far removed from the staff-resident interaction, often resulting in a mismatch (Hujala & Rissanen 2011). Caring staff in nursing homes are thus removed from the process of defining the regulatory framework of their work, from the conceptual construction of the idea of «the nursing home» and even from decisions concerning the daily operations of their nursing homes or units. On a conceptual level, then, caring staff can experience a sense of powerlessness and detachment, by not being involved in defining the premises of their work, leading to unspoken and implicit reactions to the outsiders' definition of «nursing home life», created by experts, bureaucrats, or the media. From this detachment arises *a need* in the caring staff, a need to define that which is theirs. This primary powerlessness further relates, as argued, to the development of communal sentiments that are local and strongly connected to practice; *We do, therefore **WE** are.*

As such, detachment and powerlessness relate to the need for what I argue manifests itself as *an institutional practice.* But this institutional practice develops not simply because it can and because of a sense of detachment from those above and beyond; on a more concrete level, pertaining to the specific structural framework of nursing homes, it develops *because it has to.* The context, from where the development of practice originates, including official rules, regulations and guidelines as well as the educational system, does not cover what caring staff actually have to do in everyday life. Furthermore, what is unspoken, the blanks that need to be filled in by the caring staff primarily dealing with the everyday, small decisions, is not something that is readily available to them; *it is not given and needs to be created on the spot* (Callewaert 1997: 13-25). As such, local regimes of practices develop because of *an uncertainty* relating to the specific tasks at hand.

When applied to the specific decisions caring staff make, such an uncertainty is similar to what has elsewhere been described as the professional uncertainty principle: when «standard treatment procedures» are not widely established and followed, decisions and judgment may be «highly discretionary» (Wennberg, Barnes & Zubkoff (1982) in Carter 2003a). I will add, given our context that «standard treatment procedures» are not simply missing because they have not been developed yet, but also that they cannot be widely established, given the forms of «treatment procedures» in question. The principle is seen by others as applicable to health sciences where what to do (treatment) for the healthcare provider is not given based on the premises (treatment protocols pertaining to the treatment of the condition), leading to situations where the decisions must be based on discretion rather than a previously defined «correct solution». It has been argued that the professional uncertainty principle is applicable to physicians when deciding on hospitalizations since, «at times medical conditions may lack widely established treatment protocols or clear and convincing evidence to support one treatment option over another» (Ibid.: 1179-80), leading to «a considerable level of professional discretion in deciding whether to hospitalize» (Ibid.: 1179). Elsewhere, it is argued that this principle is especially applicable to decisions concerning nursing home residents because of the high level of dementia (Gruneir et al. 2007), and that there is a general uncertainty imbedded in end-of-life treatment of elderly people (Hov et al. 2009). As such, the professional uncertainty principle is used to cover decisions about treatment options and regimens where the very effect of treatment is uncertain and where there are no protocols or guidelines assisting the decision-maker. Although primarily directed towards physicians and their decisions over the hospitalizations of nursing home residents, the principle is highly relevant and applicable also to caring staff in nursing homes.

The diffuse and unclear development of residents' illness, for instance, makes the understanding, evaluation and decisions regarding residents' well-being complicated and ambiguous. Many residents are in a more or less constant state of being eligible for hospitalization, making the decision process for the staff unclear, while being, in many cases, constant. How to relate to «the resident» is not provided those who must relate to her, and decisions concerning her are highly discretionary.

Such an understanding of the dynamics of practice in nursing homes, is contrasted not only to how practice is presented in a majority of the research literature, but also to the understanding of practice undertaken by those who train the practitioners in practice in nursing homes - nursing schools and equivalent institutions. To be brief, practice in nursing homes is presented to nursing students as abilities and techniques that are a priori (they are an inherent part of the «nursing profession», regardless of the respective nurses) and generic (they are universal), which the practitioner either has or not. Thus, it is seen to be achieved through training. Practice in nursing homes is presented and understood, therefore, as an absolute entity, similar or identical (ideally) between institutions. Neither variation nor the possibility of variation is problematized within such a perspective. Students can, if diligent, achieve mastery of such practice, and thus be a part of what is understood as the shared practice in the nursing home. Of course, such an understanding of practice has the effect of legitimizing the education at the same time. Based on such an understanding of practice, and the specific training it implies, the nursing student (registered nurse or assisting nurse) is met with a different reality in the nursing home. Against such a dominant view, Wærness argues for the importance of «*learned skills*»; the care provider is not proficient because she is an inherently «good» care provider. She must learn. Nor are the skills needed for the care provider, it is argued, part of the formal training; it is not codified (Wærness 1984, Fjær og Vabø 2013). Similarly, Davies elaborates on how the care worker is in need of acquiring practices and knowledge that are not formal:

> «*Yet there are few cases overall that could be classed in an obvious way as celebration of mastery of the principles of textbook knowledge: instead they are about weighting this knowledge against an understanding of the full circumstances of a patient, continuing to observe and puzzle when something is not quite as expected. Nurses remember with pride spotting something that others might have missed. In some instances this comes as a result of years of experience; often, however, it is a result of patient, minute and detailed observation that takes place in the sustainedly close relationship that the nurse has with the patient, and that has been singled out in this paper as the defining characteristics of caring work. (…) Instead, formal knowledge is put alongside other knowledges, leaving a considerable place for adjustment and negotiation in the light of a carefully acquired and detailed understanding of persons and situations.　The skill base for the kind of caring that is being described here has never been clearly codified.*» (Davies 1995: 22-23)

For Davies' nurse, codified knowledge and skills are not sufficient; they are not adequate to the practice which they must perform, and, consequently, need to be supplemented by other forms of knowledge and skills. Other forms of knowledge and skills relate, for the nurse, to experience and familiarity with the patient; they must be acquired. Armstrong makes a similar argument stressing that the skills required within work environments predominantly employed by women, such as care work, are not, as is often presented, inherent in those who perform them (Armstrong 2013: 258-261). Nor are the skills required inherently gendered (Ibid.). Following Wærness, Davies and Armstrong, addressing different albeit related areas, skills are not *a priori* features of the worker, nor are formal, codified skills sufficient; rather, skills are social entities acquirable through and with others through experience. The skills required «*(...) are not 'plug and play' capacities that workers bring to the job and immediately 'switch on' and use. Rather, they are like a 'flat pack': they need to be built up and integrated with the requirements of their surrounds*» (Hampson & Junor 2010: 4).

The skills required for caring staff must, in other words, be acquired through experience directly related to the precise area of their work, rather than simply through formal training or being a «good care provider». Relating to the need of acquirement, I will argue, is that such skills can only be attained with and through *others*; the skills needed to operate within the nursing home setting are inherently *shared*. The skills required in nursing homes, given the resident and given the uncertainty, are shared *because they have to be learned*. They are, at the same time, learned *because they need to be shared*. As such, *continuity*, to which we will return, can be seen as a universally relevant component of the skills required in nursing homes.

9.4. Shared practices? Continuity

Acre Woods, two episodes related to the same resident. In the large common room on a Tuesday late morning, everything is as it usually is in *the unit*: several of the residents are sitting quietly in their usual chairs or wheelchairs, not making much of a fuss, either with each other or the staff member, who occasionally walks by. The television is on, showing the regional news by the public broadcaster. As it is between meals, the room is quiet; many residents are in their rooms, while staff are busy attending to residents in their rooms or doing other tasks. Occasionally a staff member would look in, say hi or just check if everything was quiet, and then walk off again. During a period of about forty minutes, no staff member would stay in the room for longer than ten seconds. During the same period, the residents sat quietly by themselves, sometimes making short comments to a neighbor or to no one in particular, not requiring help or assistance from staff: except Pauline (see Chapter 9.6). Pauline was usually uneasy and nervous, and rarely sat quietly for too long. Today was no exception. She called out several times, a high-pitched sound, which could often be heard when walking down the corridor of the unit, almost at regular intervals, approximately five minutes between each call. Some of the residents were annoyed by this, shaking their heads, or muttering a derogatory comment, while the staff did not mind very much. Sometimes they would look in to check and tell her that everything was okay and that she could just calm down, other times no one would come. After repeating the shouts about six times every five minutes, without getting feedback from the staff, she pushed away the tray standing in front of her wheelchair. I did not make much of this, for me, insignificant action, but another resident, the lucid and well-articulated Maud, spoke out immediately, addressing me as there were no staff present: *She can´t do that, because now she can stand up!* I interpreted this as a warning about the danger of Pauline falling as she now did not have any obstacles hindering her from standing up from her wheelchair. I fetched an assisting nurse, who came immediately, re-arranged the tray and confirmed my suspicion.

Three weeks later: Pauline had fallen and broken her arm while in her room one evening. I was not present in the ward at the time, but was told by the assisting ward leader that they had *found her* shortly after, when coming in to prepare her for the evening care routine. An experienced assisting nurse had told me that it happened because *someone left her in her chair too far from her bed*, indicating that she was not able to walk the distance herself, and that the caring staff responsible should have known better. Supposedly, her arm was much better now, but some of the staff, especially the leaders, seemed anxious about a repeat event. During the preparation for the morning report meeting, most staff had already assembled, while others were finishing some minor tasks before being able to attend. Just before the start of the meeting, an assistant stopped at the entrance of the nurses´ station accompanying Pauline in her wheelchair. The assistant asked, addressing all staff members present: *Should she go into the common room or her room? NO!* the experienced assisting nurse said suddenly, raising her voice, *she shall NOT sit in her room alone. Put her in her bed!* The assistant did not respond and left. The experienced assisting nurses continued, in a calmer voice this time, addressing no one in particular: *Jesus, I don´t know how many times I´ve told people that.*

Continuity, in the form of experience and stability of staff and familiarity between staff and residents, is essential when relating to the nursing home resident. Understanding, attending and evaluating the nursing home resident is characterized by uncertainty for the caring staff. Combined, the premises of practice for caring staff result in a need to attain a set of skills that, I will argue, *needs to be learned on the spot.* Such a skill set *presupposes continuity.*

The importance of knowledge and experience extends beyond the specific residents and units, including also knowledge about and experience with the healthcare sector in general and the specific context of the respective nursing homes. Regarding decisions on hospitalization, experience in communicating with hospitals, emergency wards (in interpreting physicians´ orders, for instance), and the healthcare sector in general, proved greatly advantageous at our nursing homes. Caring staff without former experience, either with the reporting systems[5], or in communicating with unknown physicians or emergency department staff, exhibited frustration and uncertainty in coping technically and emotionally. Experience in «the sector», meanwhile, is seen as advantageous:

Conversation with on-duty registered nurse after the evening-shift described in Chapter 6.1.3, Acre Woods. After a hectic shift, the on-duty nurse reviews the events of the day over a cup of coffee. After giving her thoughts about the respective decisions she had to make during the shift, her focus drifts towards the role of the on-duty nurse and the difficulties connected to such a role. Being an on-duty nurse for the entire nursing home is a large responsibility, she explains: *But it´s also important work and you have to make difficult decisions right then and there. And you have to do it alone. Well, you´re not alone, but you have to make the decisions based on your own judgment, both about hospitalizations and other things.* Even though she has to call the emergency ward or the nursing home's physician on occasion, she says, it´s still an

---

5   Elsewhere, it has been argued that documentation relating to transfers of residents is unnecessarily time consuming, and that the information can be of little use for sender and receiver alike as the information can be perceived to be «*unreliable or irrelevant*» (McCloskey 2011). For our nursing homes, documentation connected to hospitalizations from nursing homes was not studied explicitly and in detail, as getting access to personalized information that transfer documents includes, would entail a breach of the ethical approval for the project. General approaches and perceptions towards such documentation can still be considered. Caring staff and physicians at our nursing homes considered documentation connected to hospitalization time-consuming and technically difficult. Still, they asserted that it was a necessary task, important to do correctly, and that information could be of vital importance for residents. Contrary to McCloskey's sample (consisting of one nursing home), nursing homes in our municipality use standardized electronic forms, accessible for hospitals, thus providing predictability for writer and reader, even though described as complicated. As for McCloskey's study, caring staff at our nursing homes expressed great frustration towards the amount and form of information from hospitals, explained as insufficient, confusing and/or fragmentary.

important job: *Because even though the physician has the final say, the most important thing is still how the registered nurse presents the situation to the physician. We have a lot of power! How I talk and present it, how I convey needs, has a lot to say. It will be decisive, it will determine if someone will be hospitalized or not. It´s really all about how I present it, what to include and not include. And, in the end, we are the ones who know the residents the best, usually anyway, so it´s a good thing, really. When you have been a registered nurse as long as I have, talking to physicians becomes almost like an art form. I always get my will in the end! I know how to influence, which buttons to push. And I also know the different physicians. It almost becomes like using feminine wiles[6]. You get your way in the end, one way or another. And it works every time!*

An on-duty nurse without intimate knowledge of a unit or a resident can benefit from detailed knowledge of «the system»; knowing who to contact and, more importantly, how to convey her message. Continuity can also be made relevant on an institutional level; through the communication and collaboration between institutional entities (between a nursing home and the municipality or a hospital, for instance). As seen, nursing homes from within our sample vary considerably in the form and frequency of contact with municipal representatives, while communication with hospitals has been underscored as problematic because of lack of continuity in persons of contact for nursing home staff.

In general, continuity can be seen as a significant aspect of the respective professional groups' practices, the collaboration between caring staff, and between caring staff and other professional groups. Still, most important is the caring staff's knowledge of specific residents and their experience from within their respective units.

9.4.1. Knowledge of residents

Knowledge of and experience with *specific* residents is vital for how everyday life in nursing homes evolves, for staff and residents alike. How well caring staff know the residents they tend to, how long they have known them and how long they have attended to them, is decisive for how and what happens during a day. It has been pointed out that previous knowledge and familiarity with residents (from the local community, for instance) can be decisive in securing

---

6   Translated from the Norwegian «kvinnelist».

good communication between residents and staff (Hauge 2004). I will argue that the importance of knowledge of and familiarity with residents goes beyond previous knowledge and familiarity (especially for a sample such as ours, a larger municipality), to familiarity and knowledge gained *at* the nursing homes. The significance Examples of knowledge of and experience with specific residents are many: from the trivial, to how everyday life evolves for the residents, to deciding on whether or not a resident should be hospitalized.

> Emerald Gardens. An activity worker is preparing for the activity of the day, bingo, while several caring staff members help out getting it started. Getting started proves difficult, as residents from other units are brought in, several of whom are in wheelchairs, which are difficult to maneuver in the relatively small room. The residents, most of whom are anxious to get started, wait patiently for the last remaining two residents, while the bingo equipment is set up. I sit down beside a familiar resident, ready to help her fill out the numbers on her board. The last resident arrives from another unit, brought in by an assistant, who is unfamiliar to me. The assisting nurse wheels the immobile resident towards our table, and places her close to the table so that the resident can reach the table with both hands. The assistant gets a board for the resident from another table. When she has finished, the activity worker notices the resident, walks over to her and readjusts her position, so that the resident now sits with her right side towards the table, enabling her to reach her board with her right arm. I later learn that the resident has suffered from a severe stroke, leaving her entire left side paralyzed.

This small incident could be supplemented with almost endless others; caring staff in nursing homes act and relate to residents based on residents' individual needs and preferences, not simply based on the habits of residents (cooking the egg just right), but also related to the individual somatic and cognitive needs of residents. As seen, residents are generally in a poor state, while also varying in how poor. Understanding them (literally and figuratively) and attending to their respective needs, then, implies actual knowledge and experience with *them*.

The caring staff's knowledge and experience of residents facilitates not only the physical well-being of residents, but also how they generally experience everyday life. The opposite, the lack of knowledge of and experience with residents, can lead to misunderstandings between staff and residents (overcooking the egg), and can produce more profound effects, as in the case of Pauline's fall.

Knowledge of and familiarity with residents can be said to be particularly significant for caring staff in nursing homes because of the danger of falls for residents and because of dementia among residents. Falls are not simply dangerous for residents because they can result in serious injuries, but also because of the anxiety many frail elderly experience towards the possibility of falling, or after a fall (Rubenstein et al. 1996). As such, the possibility of a fall, in addition to the experience of one, can lead to less mobility and to isolation, paradoxically increasing the possibility of falls. The potential occurrence of falls is not simply related to characteristics of the faller, but also to how her surroundings are formed and how staff members facilitate mobility and movement (Spector et al. 2007, Rubenstein et al. 1996).

Returning to our nursing homes, explicit attention to the prevention of falls varies somewhat between nursing homes; some addressed the issue often at report meetings, especially regarding specific residents, while others did not. An even greater variation is found in the mundane, everyday and often implicit attention to preventing falls. How caring staff act towards the potential dangers of falling, especially for «high-risk residents», varies greatly, not only between nursing homes, or different professional categories, but also between individual caring staff members, as seen in the excerpt with Pauline. Such variation is related to level of experience and knowledge of residents. Less experience and knowledge of residents will lead, I will argue, to a higher occurrence of falls and/or to higher use of restraints, either in the form of physical restraints, including hindering movement, and restraints through medication.

The experience and knowledge of caring staff at Acre Woods led to particular attention to the danger of falling for two residents: Rita (see Chapter 5.3) and Alice (see Chapter 10.4). For Alice, caring staff were generally concerned that her constant short walks and getting up and down from her chair would lead to a fall. For Rita, the situation was similar; she did not have much strength in her legs, but still enjoyed walking around. Caring staff, knowing Alice and Rita, paid close attention to them, or as much attention as they felt they could afford. They did not use restraints on Rita or Alice, but preferred to stay close by, supervising them whenever one of them was in the large common room. Even so, they could not prevent Rita from falling; she fell in her room, where staff members could not keep constant supervision, similar to the fall of Inga (see Chapter 6.1.2). For Rita and Alice, then, the general level of experience of the caring staff dealing directly with them, led to an increase in attention to the movement and mobility of Rita and Alice, although not sufficient to prevent Rita from falling. For Alexandra (see Chapter 6.2) *inexperience* and *lack of knowledge* about her, led, in my opinion, to her falling; an assistant not familiar with her left her unattended while seated in a way not deemed proper by more experienced caring staff.

Similar to dealing with potential falls, experience and knowledge is, I will argue, a prerequisite for understanding and generally dealing with residents suffering from dementia. Residents suffering from dementia are demanding and complicated; experience and knowledge not only of dementia but also of the specific residents suffering from dementia are vital for their well-being in nursing homes.

Residents suffering from dementia pose significant challenges for caring staff, especially in somatic units. These challenges are primarily, but not solely, connected to difficulties in communication and language, consequently also in *understanding* the residents. Relating to such challenges, residents suffering from dementia as a «group» (a problematic term), are at times considered a burden, for instance «put to bed» earlier than other residents. Furthermore, the challenges connected to residents suffering from dementia might influence, it has been argued, decisions of hospitalizations, as «(...) *the complexity of care*» places «(...) *an additional onus on nursing staff to identify changing health conditions and act accordingly*» (Gruneir et al. 2007: 447). Residents suffering from dementia pose difficult and significant challenges for caring staff, potentially leading them to be hospitalized more frequently, or simply differently, than other residents. As such, «(...) *familiarity with the sequelae of dementia disease and related disorders*», is pointed out as significant for adequate approaches to residents suffering from dementia (Ibid.: 454). Knowledge of and experience with the disease of dementia, its development and its effect on residents, is essential for the caring staff's approaches to residents.

I will argue that experience with and knowledge of *specific residents* suffering from dementia is significant, in addition to that of the disease and its development in itself. Residents suffering from dementia are influenced by the disease in different ways, at different stages, leading to different needs and different approaches from the caring staff. As seen from the excerpt of the reading of the newspaper, Leif and Constance had entirely different perceptions of the situation, and different skill sets in dealing with each other and others.

Dementia for them was not simply a matter of being at different stages of a development, but also of *form*. For Constance, her particular form of dementia had the effect of her not «finding her place» in the unit (see Chapter 8.4); she did not fit in: not with the staff, with the «clear» residents, or with the «forgetful» residents. Ida (Chapter 8.2.2), further illustrates the difficulties in understanding and interpreting residents suffering from dementia: apparently lucid and well-functioning, but still «lost at sea».

A generic understanding of the disease, I will argue, does not suffice in dealing with its various forms. Facilitating the activities of Leif and Constance demands specific knowledge of and experience with them, rather than dementia in general. Understanding Ida's challenges, similarly, presupposes former experience with *her*. Calming Cate also presupposed knowledge of her, but also familiarity; the familiar hand could sooth her, while, I will argue, only the experienced hand would find her. Attending and addressing residents with dementia, then, requires detailed and intimate knowledge of and experience with the respective residents, in addition to formal and generic knowledge of the disease. The same applies when deciding whether or not hospitalization is a beneficial course of action for residents suffering from dementia; interpreting nuances in body-language (for a resident not able to verbally communicate), for instance, can be pivotal in assessing a complex situation with uncertain outcomes.

9.4.2. Experience from within the unit

Knowledge of and experience from within the unit is, as seen, an important aspect of nursing home life. The unit, rather than the entire nursing home, can be the entity towards which the identification of caring staff is directed. Units are also, albeit to a varying degree, the premise for organizing everyday life. Knowledge of and experience with the respective units of work, therefore, might be more significant than experience in nursing homes in general or even other units at the same nursing home:

Conversation with an assisting nurse on an evening-shift during the weekday at a medium sized private nursing home, the United States. At about 20.00, a female assisting nurse is cleaning the kitchen area, alone in the unit. All but two residents, who are sitting quietly in front of the television, have retired to their rooms, while no other staff members are in sight. After some «light» conversation, I ask her about the work schedule for the unit. She explains that she only works late shifts, from 14 to 22. What days she works and the number of days per week differ from week to week. When asked about how common such arrangement are, she replies that it varies a lot from staff member to staff member, but that this is the best solution for her, because of studies she has to attend during the day. Although this poses problems for her, having two small children, she has no other choice, she explains. When asked if she works in the unit exclusively, she responds that she primarily works on this floor, the dementia unit, but that she sometimes is told to work in other places as well: *This is very common too; everyone has to work in different places.* I ask her if she would prefer to change units regularly or to stay in «her» unit exclusively: *No, I don't like it. It is harder to work on other floors. Some of the residents there are, you know… more difficult. And we don't know them, so it takes longer. And they don't get to know us either. So, it doesn't work so well. It would be better just to work in one place.* We continue our conversation by discussing the differences between the respective units. The assisting nurse emphasizes again that she prefers her unit as she is familiar with it, but also that it is «easier» in the unit in general: *In the evening, it is usually easy here. Very calm. In other places, not so much. But suddenly they will come walking down the hallway, so you have to be ready all the time. But here at least I know them.»*

Working sporadically in other units had led the assisting nurse to appreciate not only her work in her primary unit, but also the significance of experience from within the unit. Perhaps her sporadic meeting with other units left her more capable of appreciating such importance. Still, I will argue, the significance of the unit, of experience from within it, does not merely arise from the need to «belong to a place», but also from the need to master complex and multifaceted everyday life:

A casual conversation with three assisting nurses during their lunch break, Durmstrang. After a while, the conversation drifts towards levels of staffing in the unit: *It can be very demanding if a lot of things happen at the same time. And they are really different, right, the residents I mean, so different things happen with different residents. So we have to be good at planning then and there. One resident would like to have her morning routines one way, a second another way, a third, and so on. In addition, one day might also be different from another. Perhaps you don't want to get up that day, perhaps you have a bad morning, perhaps it would be best not to get her up at all that day.*

Knowledge of and experience from within the respective units is not simply significant because that happens to be the place where residents are, but also because of the general organizational centrality of the unit in nursing. As seen from a typical day at the nursing home: caring staff *must have* knowledge of the unit to cope with the work of everyday life. Everyday life of the nursing home is routinized on the level of the unit; the experienced staff member falls into the rhythm of the routines, while the neophyte tries to adapt. Routines then *presuppose knowledge of and experience from within the unit*. The significance of specific knowledge of and experience from within the unit is still varied, as is the function of the unit, specifically how it is organized in relation to the rest of the nursing home. However, the significance of specific knowledge of and experience from within the unit is generally accentuated by the instability of the workforce, a universal point for our nursing homes. The high prevalence of sick leave and consequent high (although different) use of temporary staff, leaves some units at some times «understaffed». For those who remain, or for those who have to cope with the supervision of inexperienced staff in addition to demanding residents, knowledge of and experience from their respective units become essential. The staffing levels in units might vary, adding to the general perception of the toil in the nursing home, between nursing homes, between units in a nursing home, and between different shifts and weekdays in the same unit. Again: knowledge of and experience from within the unit can become essential not only in general, but particularly at certain times.

9.4.3. Continuity and hospitalization

Continuity is significant for small and large matters: for the ability to adjust to the everyday routines of nursing home life, and to help a resident get the preferred spread on a piece of bread just right. Continuity *of* caring staff is significant for residents and for caring staff. It is, I will argue, especially significant when coping with exceptional incidents breaking with the familiar, sudden decisions on whether or not to hospitalize, for instance. In such situations, where the uncertainty is fundamental, caring staff and/or physicians, sometimes in mutual collaboration, sometimes separately, have to make decisions based not on precise knowledge of the potential outcome or on formal knowledge, but on former experience. Continuity, in the form of knowledge of and experience with specific residents is also significant when caring for the many residents who are in a more or less constant state of being poorly or ill. Many decisions about hospitalization and treatment are not episodic, as we have seen, but constant and perpetually difficult. Knowing the resident, in such cases (which really is not a case, but rather the norm), is essential, for instance regarding interpreting small changes in the state of a confused resident who has difficulty in communicating verbally. Experienced caring staff at our nursing homes convey the ability to sense small changes in frail residents, as one assisting nurse stated: It was in her eyes. Similarly, Phillips´ (et al. 2006) care assistants say that they have the ability to notice subtle changes in their residents, much as a mother does with a sick child.

Continuity is influential for what can be described as universal dynamics at play at all nursing homes. As seen, informal recognition and position for caring staff in the units can be gained by experience; by being knowledgeable about routines and of residents, or simply by knowing what to do. Such traits can, on occasion, surpass that of formal authority; an assisting nurse intimately familiar with the unit can influence others, implicitly and explicitly, in ways that the formal authority of the inexperienced registered nurse cannot. Inexperienced caring staff might be inclined to follow the lead of the experienced assisting nurse, consciously or not, by being shown, deliberately or not, how to perform.

Continuity is also universally relevant for nursing homes because of «*the hardship and toil*» *of the nursing home* and *the nursing home resident.* The level of staffing in nursing homes combined with the workload connected to the nursing home resident, leads to an experience of hardship and difficulty for the caring staff member. Coping with having a small number of colleagues (especially on certain days or times of day), and residents who are frail and reliant on constant assistance, presuppose knowledge and experience. Knowing what to do, when and how, leaves the caring staff member with coping tools for a strenuous everyday life. As seen in examples where caring staff do not possess experience and knowledge, the work burden increases, for the inexperienced *and* for the experienced, affecting also the routines and potential well-being of residents. The universal need for experience and knowledge is accentuated by the lack of formal rules and guidelines, manageable by the development of routines and institutional practices by experienced caring staff, and adopted by others.

While such a dynamic is universal for all nursing homes in the sense of providing premises to which all nursing homes must relate, the outcome of the dynamic is not given by the premises. The need for experience and knowledge to cope with the perceived «hardship and toil» and an uncertainty is shared, while *how experience and knowledge manifest themselves in practices is not.* While the need for continuity can be seen as universal for all nursing homes, the actual level of continuity can explain variation between them.

9.5. Towards an institutional practice

Nursing homes, and even units within a nursing home, *develop distinct, unique and internally shared sets of practices.* Such sets or regimes of practices can be labelled *the institutional practice,* designating a specificity in time and space. The institutional practice is *internally shared,* although being implicit and unofficial, and not necessarily equal to that of the institutional practice of others.

How can this be? I argue that regimes of practices are generated in nursing homes and nursing home units because it must; because the premises caring staff must relate to necessitate the creation of local and informal regimes of practices. These premises, most notably the rules that govern nursing homes, the state of «the nursing home resident» and the workload and content of work for caring staff, create a fundamental uncertainty for caring staff pertaining to large and small tasks and decisions alike. Such uncertainty further contributes to local rather than generic understandings and actions; they are not provided from «the outside». Thus arises the need for an institutional practice.

Let us trace back and elaborate on this argument, starting with the premises for caring staff: the rules and routines. «Rules» work, it has been argued, when they are respected and deemed adequate for the area they are intended to cover (Goffman 1971[7] - see also Bourdieu 2012). The rules of the nursing home can be viewed as inefficient at times, in part because of unintended consequences, in part because they are inadequate in form and scope. When rules are not deemed appropriate or adequate to the area they are supposed to cover, they can be opposed, altered, or added to. Such oppositions and/or resistance have

---

[7]   *«Rules are effective (insofar as they are) because those to whom they apply believe them to be right and come to conceive of themselves both in terms of who and what it is that compliance allows them to be, and in terms of what deviation implies they have become. The sanctioning system associated with a rule is effective (insofar as it is) because it proclaims the individual's success or failure at realizing what he and others feel he should be, and, more abstractly, proclaims the individual's compliance with or deviation from rules in general».* (Goffman 1971: 98)

implications on a theoretical and a practical level - for the researcher and for the practitioner. On a theoretical level, the potential inadequacy of rules implies that rules and patterns, generally speaking, do not necessarily give an apt description of what agents actually do (Prieur & Sestoft 2006: 30-31). The researcher cannot base descriptions of action or practice solely on formal, descriptive patterns of intention. For the practitioner, and more importantly in this context, rules and patterns do not necessarily work as determinant directives for practice (Ibid., Bourdieu 2012).

For the rules of the nursing home, agents do resist and oppose them, not necessarily with intent or deliberation, but because they are not experienced as being adequate or sufficient for everyday practice. Rules, then, can contribute to a sense of detachment and powerlessness for the caring staff. Consequently, rules at the nursing home will be manipulated, opposed, altered or ignored. Primarily, however, they will be altered and supplemented locally, because they can be inadequate for those who are supposed to implement them. Rules provide *a space from which practice can be formed*, rather than determining it.

The form of rules and regulations contributes to uncertainty for caring staff. This uncertainty is accentuated by the variation of residents´ needs and capabilities, and experiences of toil for caring staff. Combined, these elements constitute a *fundamental uncertainty* for caring staff; the tasks, actions and function of caring staff are not given or even provided, but must be developed and implemented locally. The blanks that need to be filled in by the caring staff, are not something that is readily available to them; *it is not given and need to be created on the spot*. As such, an institutional practice develops *because* of a fundamental uncertainty.

Nursing home units have been used in this chapter to illustrate both the need for and the formative mechanics of an institutional practice. Units can differ within the same nursing home because collective identity and sense of community is placed on the level of units, generating different and differing institutional practices. Nursing homes with a clear division of units, such as Acre Woods, can and will produce different and unique institutional practices in their respective units.

However, caring staff do not come unequipped when facing this fundamental uncertainty. The uncertainty can, in part, be tamed by experience and familiarity, most notably by detailed and intimate knowledge about residents. In the ongoing process of creating and recreating practices, experience and knowledge - among caring staff, with residents, with the nursing homes and with the unit - is essential not only as a coping mechanism, but also for developing and implementing that which is not explicit.

In conclusion, nursing homes, and even units within a nursing home, *develop distinct, unique and internally shared sets of practices - the institutional practice – all the while relating to the same dynamic of developing them, primarily in the form of incentives to create a community* (sometimes within a community), *and to make sense of that which is not immediately apparent.* The institutional practice is functional and pragmatic; it is adequate to the area in which it is implemented. The understanding of the institutional practice is derived from the theory of the practical sense (see Chapter 10), but is also an adaptation of it; the institutional practice is (more strongly) bounded in space, local with relatively distinct boundaries from other institutional practices, as evident in different units at the same nursing home. Regardless of differences in form of the institutional practice, it *shares a dynamic of creation.*

9.6. Meeting a resident: knowing Pauline

While most incidents concerning acute illness and the potential of hospitalization can be analyzed in connection to various forms of interrelated factors, some incidents seem unrelated to factors such as staffing level, treatment options and competence in the unit. Perhaps their occurrence is not to be explained by underlying factors. However, I will argue that *continuity* relates to most such incidents, even the ones seemingly unrelated. For the non-hospitalization of Pauline, knowledge of and experience with Pauline's former illness and her wishes for treatment regimens were taken, perhaps implicitly, under consideration.

Pauline

Pauline was anxious and uneasy, not finding peace with «nursing home life» or in her unit (see also excerpt with Pauline in the introduction to this chapter). She was bound to a wheelchair, but could move swiftly around in her wheelchair, and did so, often to the annoyance of caring staff members. On one occasion, Pauline was nowhere to be found when she was supposed to receive her medication, later to be discovered in the activity center on a different floor, alone.

Apparently, she had taken the staff elevator by herself, although no one could understand how she had managed. *Well it's not the first time and will probably not be the last time. Typical!* another resident said after overhearing the turn of events from staff members talking among themselves. Generally, Pauline was considered «difficult» by most of the caring staff, not because she needed excessive care, but rather because she did not always comply; she would often answer disrespectfully, if at all, and seldom did as asked.

The end came swiftly for Pauline, and when it came, the caring staff, despite their strained relationship, tried their best to comfort and take care of Pauline.

Two assisting nurses and I are enjoying a short break in the nurses' station shortly after breakfast on a Friday when the assisting unit leader arrives, more flustered than her usual stoic self. She explains that Pauline has still not got out of bed (Pauline was usually an early riser, and her sleeping in had already been mentioned at the morning report meeting): *Perhaps it's another drip*, she says, concerned. The assisting unit leader says that she has called the physician and that he is on his way.

About forty minutes later the physician has already been to see Pauline. The assisting nurse informs me: *He believes the same as me, a drip might have affected the center of sleep.* The assisting unit leader explains that she believes that there was nothing they could have done differently, *I believe, because she had a precondition leaving her vulnerable for drips and other things. Normally you only live with* [name of the disease] *for 5 or 6 years, but she has lived with it for 13, so...* The assisting unit leader dismisses the idea of Pauline's sleeping in being connected to medication: *We have checked.* All in all, the assisting unit leader acknowledged that even though it has only been a short while, she has come to terms with the end getting closer for Pauline: *There is only so little they can do now. Whatever happens, happens, and there is no point in hospitalizing now. They cannot do anything more now.* She seemed adamant that staying in her room in the unit is the best thing for Pauline now, and that she might not have much time left. Because of this she has already called and informed the next of kin, who are on their way.

The following Monday morning a table stands in the corridor outside what used to be Pauline's room. A picture of Pauline stands on it next to a burning candle. Pauline died Sunday night, her family present. The assisting unit leader is already planning for the arrival of the next resident.

Variation in hospitalization

Nursing homes and/or units develop institutional practices, meanwhile all sharing a dynamic of how and why they are generated. But how does an institutional practice relate to practices of hospitalization? And more importantly in this context: how can we explain differences in practices of hospitalization?

In this concluding chapter, I will argue that practices of hospitalization to a large degree are *embedded within an institutional practice*. Many decisions regarding hospitalization share the general features described for the institutional practice; concrete procedures are not present, outcomes are unclear – uncertainty prevails. Decisions of hospitalization relate, as a part of the institutional practice, to a local regime of «how things are done» – nursing homes and even nursing home units develop these regimes *differently*. As such, variation in the practices of hospitalization occurs.

This argument will be elaborated on in three parts in this chapter. First, I will revisit the discussion about influencing factors for hospitalization given in Chapter 5. I will argue that isolated factors do not sufficiently explain practices of hospitalization, and that even apparently determinant factors can have a more ambiguous effect, leaving the explanations presented in much of the research literature somewhat insufficient. Secondly, I will present a theoretical foundation for my argument. Bourdieu's theory of the practical sense will be presented, not with the aim of explaining or «proving» the institutional practice, but with the aim of further understanding how it can be that caring staff act as they do. It will be argued that caring staff share the dynamic of the practical sense when developing an institutional practice. Finally, and based on this theoretical exploration, I will attempt to explain in more detail how variation in hospitalization between nursing homes occurs. Two important and under-communicated aspects will be highlighted: differences in interaction with family and differences in collaboration with physicians. These elements are a) more significant than those argued for in the majority of research, b) integrated in an institutional practice and most importantly c) can explain differences in practices of hospitalization.

10.1. The interplay of factors revisited: effects on hospitalization

To what do decisions on hospitalizations in nursing homes relate? What are the influencing factors, and *how* do they influence? Moving from a discussion about the institutional practice in general, we are better equipped to analyze how factors can influence the specific practice of hospitalization. Meanwhile, an analysis of the specific practice of hospitalization can add to our understanding of practice in general. In this sub-chapter, conditions of particular and potential significance for practices of hospitalization will be revisited.

I will argue, in a continuation of the discussion given in Chapter 5, that the connection or relationship between conditions and outcome - hospitalization - is individual, involved and changing: «*Nursing homes, like the rest of the healthcare system, are complex adaptive institutions, and it is likely that these apparently contradictory associations may be explained by unmeasured factors producing confounding effects*» (McGregor et al. 2014: 9). The way in which conditions relate to each other, to the structural framework, and to practices of hospitalization, does not necessarily follow a distinct pattern, and when it does, or rather when it is presented as such, there might be more to the pattern than what is immediately visible. Patterns of influence should be understood as being composed in an intricate, non-determinant way; that is, a given factor does not influence the outcome regardless of other factors. A simplification of our understanding of modes of influence can be illustrated in a model, also serving as an elaboration of the model presented in Chapter 5. Again, the model will serve as an illustration and is not meant to be understood literally. The model does highlight how factors can be mutually *and* relatively significant. Note also that now we have moved from the general term *practice*, to the more specific and delimited term *institutional practice*.

A model does not sufficiently capture the complexity of the potential variation of influence, unfortunately. The relationship between certain institutional conditions (such as size of nursing home) and outcomes (such as rates of hospitalization) can, for instance, be *spurious*. To analyze such relationships, we need to deconstruct what factors are at play (and not), to analyze their respective relationship to one another, and to analyze how they relate, individually or collectively, to outcomes. The process of analyzing such relationships resembles the act of peeling an onion, although for us, there are several different onions, each unique, with different numbers and qualities within its layers.

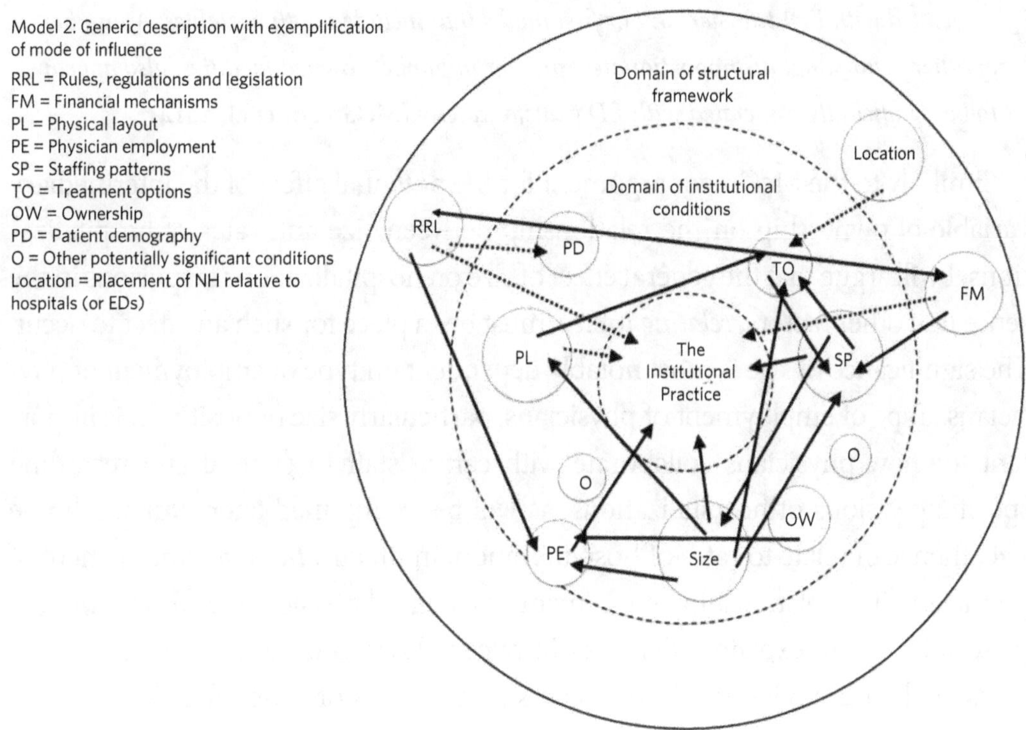

10.1.1. The spuriousness of size

«Spurious effects» are understood as connections that are seemingly strong and direct, and might be presented as such in research literature where the connection between an isolated factor or a set of factors and the outcome appears determinant, but proves coincidental and/or weaker than previously assumed when the onion is further peeled. Spurious effects are, in other words, connections between factors or between conditions and outcome that are not, strictly speaking, causal (A does not determine B, but A may influence B, given C, D, E and F). *Size of nursing homes* can serve as perhaps the best example of the production of spurious effects on rates of hospitalizations. Size is, in research literature, often pointed out as having the strongest effect on rates of hospitalizations for all factors included. Only exceptionally does analysis problematize the apparent direct and respective effect of size:

> «*The bivariate association between facility size and a lower rate of transfer is likely confounded by the disproportionate distribution of large facilities across public ownership. This is supported by the fact that facility size was not found to be significantly*

associated with ED[1] transfers in our first model that included both variables. A number of other factors, not disproportionately present in publicly owned facilities, also appear to be significantly associated with ED transfer rates.» (McGregor et al. 2014)

Similarly to the McGregor argument for the potential effect of the intermediary variable of ownership on the relationship between size and rates of hospitalizations, I will argue that the general effect of size on hospitalizations is spurious in the sense that other factors, *relating to size*, must be in place for such an effect to occur. The significance of size is most notably dependent on type of employment of physicians. Type of employment of physicians, particularly size of positions, is important for how physicians collaborate with caring staff in general and regarding specific decisions of hospitalizations, as will be exemplified later. Nursing home size, then, can relate to rates of hospitalization, indirectly, *through* employment of physicians. The relationship between employment of physicians and rates of hospitalization could explain differences in rates of hospitalization in a more precise manner than the relationship between size and rates of hospitalizations, but, as seen in the next sub-chapter, also this connection is not as straightforward as it might seem. To return to nursing home size: it is not size in itself, but the relationship between size and type of employment of physicians (which may or may not be influenced by nursing home size) that has a more direct effect on decisions of hospitalization. Slagsvold made a similar argument analyzing the connection between size and *«quality of care»*. Size, in itself, does not determine differences between small and large nursing homes in quality of care, rather other attributes *related* to being large or small are seen as decisive (1986).

For the analysis of practice, if only the more or less direct effect of separate factors is included, effect can be exaggerated. Spurious effects, such as in the example presented, might cover an effectual relationship that is sporadic and varied, as evident when analyzing a broader spectrum of relevant, interrelated factors.

10.1.2. The sporadic effect of staffing level and physical layout

Sporadic effects are taken to mean connections and relationships between factors that are flexible, changing and varied, both in time (within a nursing

---

1   Emergency department.

home, for instance) and space (between nursing homes within the same area, for instance). The very nature of sporadic effects makes them difficult to grasp and convey, making analyses of them similar to that of spurious effects; they are often presented as less complex than they are. To complicate matters further, the sporadic effects of relevant factors on practices of hospitalization can be related both to *degree of effect*, in time and space and to *type or direction of effect*. What affects what?

Size, in itself, produces spurious effects on practice in nursing homes; the influence is dependent on additional factors, employment of physicians, among others. I will further argue that even when including physician employment, the influence (size → physician employment → practice) is varied and non-determinant. Larger nursing homes do, generally speaking, offer closer to full-time positions to physicians than smaller nursing homes, often exceeding the minimum requirement given by the municipality. Larger and medium-sized nursing homes are also more inclined to employ physicians directly, rather than through the municipality. Private nursing homes, meanwhile, are also more inclined to employ physicians independently, as opposed to public ones, but not necessarily in larger positions, making a potential connection between *ownership*, size and physician employment, in addition to size and employment. However, and regardless of these potential connections, the mode of physician employment is, like size, still not a decisive factor *in itself*, for practices of hospitalizations; rather it is through its relationship to the *forms of collaboration* between physician and caring staff that the mode of employment is effectual. As will be elaborated on, this connection seems to be significant: physicians employed in or close to full-time positions *are* better integrated in the work environment than others are. However, the collaboration between physicians and caring staff, particularly the integration of the physician within the caring staff environment, evolves differently at different nursing homes, and also within a nursing home. As such, modes of employment for physicians and the consequent decisions that are based on the collaboration between physician and staff, relate differently to size, on the one hand, and practice, on the other, making the connection, although seemingly strong, non-determinant.

How the physical layout of nursing homes influences practice, can serve as another example of potential sporadic influences. Physical layout, understood as the physical environment of nursing homes, consists both of the interior physical appearance of nursing homes and to the subtler atmosphere. The physical layout of nursing homes might relate to ownership, in the sense that private nursing homes have more autonomy over their physical space than public nursing homes. Physical layout, in combination with ownership, also relates strongly to size of nursing homes, as we have seen, for obvious and less obvious reasons. Of particular importance is the relationship between physical layout, size and ownership on the one hand, and the organization of units in nursing homes, including level and form of unit autonomy, on the other. Physical layout, ownership and size, combined and respectively, also influence staffing patterns. Nursing homes might have to adjust staffing patterns based on physical layout, private nursing homes have, overall, a different composition of caring staff than public ones, while staffing patterns - particularly for registered nurses and physicians - are strongly influenced by size of nursing home.

These are but a few of the potential connections between physical layout, differing conditions and practice that could be drawn. These will still suffice to illustrate the dynamics of influence: physical layout does influence practice in nursing homes more or less directly, but its primary influence on practice depends on other factors, which are different for each nursing home. It is through and in combination with other factors, most notably ownership, size and staffing patterns, that physical layout influences practice. This connection, *works differently at different times and places*, making the effect *sporadic*. The effect between physical layout and practice can be described as sporadic in the sense that it is dependent on the specific qualities of each inter-related relevant factor: *by altering the qualities of one of these factors, the effect also changes*. To simplify for illustrative purposes: the effect of physical layout on the practice of two nursing homes with more or less identical physical layout, size and ownership, will most likely be different if staffing patterns (in the form of having an in-house physician, or not, or having more experienced assisting nurses, or not) differ. Such a difference can be illustrated, yet again somewhat simplistically, in a model highlighting only the above-mentioned factors and their potential respective influence in two hypothetical nursing home settings (illustrated both by significance of institutional condition (size of circle) and influence (type of arrow).

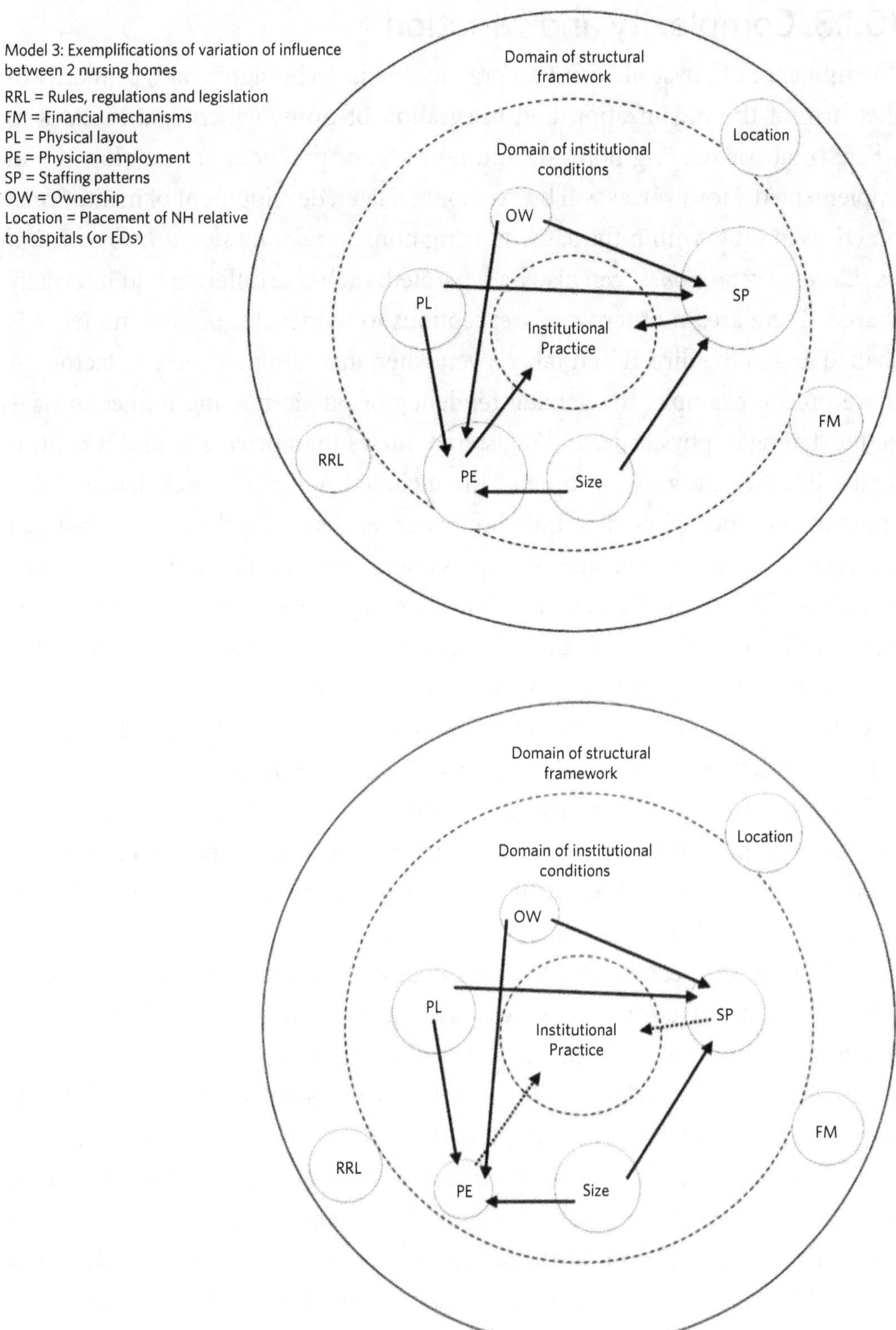
Model 3: Exemplifications of variation of influence between 2 nursing homes
RRL = Rules, regulations and legislation
FM = Financial mechanisms
PL = Physical layout
PE = Physician employment
SP = Staffing patterns
OW = Ownership
Location = Placement of NH relative to hospitals (or EDs)
Domain of structural framework
Domain of institutional conditions
Location
OW
SP
PL
Institutional Practice
FM
RRL
PE
Size
Domain of structural framework
Domain of institutional conditions
Location
OW
SP
PL
Institutional Practice
FM
RRL
PE
Size

10.1.3. Complexity and variation

The influence of physical layout on practice seems to be significant, primarily in the form of the organization and integration of units, which again relates to *where* (units or nursing homes?) and *how* sets of practices are developed and implemented. However, as will be exemplified later, development of institutional practices in units within the same nursing home – *relating similarly to identical institutional conditions* – can also be separated; each one different and internally shared. There are, in other words, exceptions to tendencies of how influence is shaped and to the direction it takes, even when including a variety of factors. A more precise example: the general tendency of public nursing homes to have better staffing of physicians and registered nurses than private homes is contradicted in different ways by some of the included nursing homes. Durmstrang chose to offer their physician more hours per resident than the average, but had less registered nurses' hours per residents than average. Galactic Manor prioritized differently, having far beyond the average registered nurses' hours per resident, while only the minimum physician hours per resident. As such, the relationship between variables can be described not only as sporadic in the sense of shifting in time and place, but also *in how the influence is directed*. The identical relationship between identical factors might generate different outcomes in different nursing homes. The two nursing homes closest to one another in formal features and characteristics related similarly to similar institutional conditions, but they are on opposite sides of the spectrum of coverage of full-time positions per resident when including all nursing homes.

Staffing patterns can be said to be more directly influential on practice, than other influential factors mentioned, such as size and physical layout. That being said, analyzing the more or less direct influence of staffing patterns on practice is, though alluring, problematic for two reasons. First, the staffing pattern is not created from a vacuum; it is affected by other factors in addition to being effectual. Second, the more or less direct effect of staffing pattern on practice cannot be understood simply by describing its general qualities or, as is the case for treatment options, simply by occurrence (how many and at what time, for instance). It must also incorporate informal traits of caring staff, most notably experience and continuity of care between staff and residents. To understand the difference in influence and effect between the mentioned factors and practice, we need to move beyond the formal qualities of the object of study and ask: what is it *about* staffing patterns that generates difference?

10.1.4. The study of variation: serendipitous patterns

The effect of potentially relevant factors on practice can be spurious and sporadic, difficult to grasp. Giving credence to trends and tendencies, for the researcher, can, however alluring, be problematic and even misleading. The problem of measuring effect is also connected to scale. Larger studies, seen in detail, tend only to include a few relevant factors and only seldom analyze how factors are interrelated, thus producing findings that exaggerate the effects of one or a few factors. A study of our sample, meanwhile, is also problematic especially for purposes of generalizations and universality (as discussed in Chapter 1). But a small sample, such as ours, can also reveal exceptions to (apparent) patterns not visible when including a large sample, exceptions that can reveal the more or less (at least seemingly) coincidental connection between factors. Such exceptions are not only relevant for their intrinsic value, but might also challenge inferences made on behalf of a larger sample.

Physicians' individualized approach to treatment of residents can serve as an example. Physicians in nursing homes can have very different approaches to their role in nursing homes, sometimes to the point of physicians going well beyond the tasks they are obliged to perform.

> Medium sized, private non-profit nursing home, Canada, evening-shift. A physician exits the room of a resident, entering directly into the large common room. He has blood splatters all over his shirt and appears to be somewhat agitated. He approaches us[2], asks who we are, and introduces himself as a physician, before explaining a procedure he has just done in one of the residents' rooms.

> He has just completed his rounds, being scheduled for an afternoon shift in the unit. The resident he attended to had a blood clot in the knee, which he, alone, proceeded to drain while in the room of the resident, he explains. He did so, he says, even though *it is a hospital procedure*. He chooses to do procedures like that himself, he continues, because *that's just who I am*. Later he talks about why he did so; he says that he likes to *go the extra mile* for the residents, so he knows that the resident will be better after the procedure. It takes him 30 minutes, while going to the hospital, getting it performed, and coming back would take much longer. He says that is it is his choice to do

---

2   On fieldwork in the nursing homes from our international sample, researchers worked in pairs.

more than what he is obliged to do. *And they appreciate it* he explains, *she gives me hugs and kisses.* He looks at an assisting nurse to get confirmation, which he gets.

He gives the impression of being very dedicated, of going out of his way to take care of elders in need, and points out several times that the tasks he performs are beyond what he is obliged to do. Since he has no social life, as he explains it, his visits have become his social life, and he *uses them* to prepare himself for his own retirement.

Later, he explains that he sees the bureaucracy connected to his work as too demanding and hindering his work. If he were to do what he *is supposed to do*, he says, relating primarily to the forms and amount of paperwork and documentation, *I would do far less than what I am actually doing.* He explains that he is sloppy with his paperwork, especially for less serious matters, while no one can complain about what he does for the more serious cases. He proceeds to give an example of how he can «bypass» the system in certain instances and get medication from the emergency ward, as he has done tonight, to bring help more swiftly and efficiently to residents. He produces a vial from his pocket, with some form of medicine.

Practices of hospitalization at a nursing home (or unit) are strongly connected to the preferences of physicians, either in the form of explicit preferences and approaches (such as the above example) or by not taking an explicit stance, and thus elevating the potential influence of caring staff and/or families. While the significance of physicians' preferences on variation of practice of hospitalization will be revisited shortly, for now the example can illustrate how physicians' approaches can be influential within a small sample such as ours.

Within such a small sample, the potential influence of a single resident on institutional rates of hospitalization also becomes evident. At two of the smaller nursing homes within the sample, *one* respective resident accounted for a large percentage of the respective nursing home's hospitalizations. For one of the nursing homes, one single resident, suffering from a rare blood disease resulting in him going regularly to the hospital, amounted to more than half of the nursing home's annual hospitalizations. While some of the transfers of the resident in question can be labelled as «appointments» or «check-ups», a majority of them were not, and would, by most standards, be labelled as «acute». Being a small nursing home, the single resident elevated the overall annual rate of hospitalization for the nursing home, leading also to a high relative rate of hospitalization for the nursing home. Were it not for that single resident, the nursing home would have compared significantly differently to other nursing homes regarding institutional rates of hospitalization.

The examples mentioned speak to a point often missing from research literature (again, related to the relatively large samples of most studies); the relationship between variables, for specific institutions, might be confounding and non-generalizable. That is not to say that they are coincidental - there are reasons behind the relationship - but rather that complex relationships discussed cannot be easily generalized for all nursing homes within a sample. The influence of the irregularities mentioned could, I will argue, contribute to understanding *the underlying and generalizable structural relationships between factors and practice*, not to be confused with the determining effect of the occurrence of a quality of a factor on practice.

Long-term bed nursing homes within a small geographical area with similar patient groups exhibit varied practices. Practices vary formally and informally, for specific, measurable practices (such as the occurrence of hospitalization) and for more general, unmeasurable practices (such as the collaboration between caring staff and physicians, and interaction with family, for instance). This variation is rooted in an institutional practice. The variation in institutional practice, leads to, I will argue shortly, variations in practices of hospitalization. But from where is that which in the first place is varied, the institutional practice, generated?

10.2. The institutional practice and variation

To understand variation of practice, so we can understand variation of practices of hospitalizations, we must revisit our general understanding of practice, theoretically and how it can be applied specifically to the nursing home context.

10.2.1. The practical sense

Revising a theoretical understanding, based on Bourdieu's theory of practice, including the interdependency between practice, habitus and structure, we can start with the more general aspects of how practice can be understood, briefly dwell on how practice relates to structure and agency, ending up with how the theory of practice can contribute to an analysis of variation.

First, and on a fundamental level, man lives his life according to rhythms. To do one's job as a man, according to Bourdieu, implies a degree of conformity to a social order. Man must respect rhythms, to keep on track and not fall out of line: «*the fundamental virtue of conformity*» (Bourdieu 2012: 161). We do not simply adjust to rhythms out of comfort, but also because it is demanded, in the form of a «*submission to collective rhythms*» (Ibid.). Adapting to the collective rhythm is not simply an external representation of the collective, but forms the very foundation of the structure from which the group is created. As such, practice has an inherent *collective* component.

Implicitly we can surmise that practice, by a Bourdieuan understanding, somehow relates to «rules» (in the sense of «that which governs beyond the contemplations of individuals or groups», rather than «rules» as specific schemes of management, as discussed earlier). This relationship, as Bourdieu presents it, is complex and imprecise. Practice, in itself, is not absolutely governed or determined by rules, nor do they follow distinct patterns, as exemplified in an early study of marriage patterns in Kabyle. Bourdieu found, to summarize, that the logic of marriage was more complex than what a structuralistic analysis would convey (Bourdieu 2012: 30-31, Prieur & Sestoft 2006: 31). The structuring forces, in the form of rules of marriages, were not necessarily followed *even though they are presented as such*. Patterns and models can be constructed (by the agent and the researcher, although the latter should be careful in doing so), but practice does not follow mechanically from them, nor can they be derived from them by the researcher[3]. Practice cannot, in other words, be deduced from the models often used to describe them. Practice, relating for instance to the exchange of gifts, should be read as encompassing a level of strategy (although not in the sense of «rational man»), rather than being strictly in compliance with rules. Alternatives exist for Bourdieu's agent; practice is not, strictly speaking, determined. Still, the actions of the agent cannot be understood simply based on deliberations and consciousness. Rather, the

---

3   This general point has been illustrated both by the mentioned analysis of marriage practices in Kabyle and in Bourdieu's criticism of Marcell Mauss´ interpretation of «the gift». The reciprocity of the gift-exchange, argues Bourdieu, is presented as adhering to rigid models:

> *«Cycles of reciprocity», mechanical interlockings of obligatory practices, exists only for the absolute gaze of the omniscient, omnipresent spectator, who, thanks to his knowledge of the social mechanics, is able to be present at the different stages of the «cycle». In reality, the gift may be unreciprocated, when one obliges an ungrateful person: in may be rejected as an insult, inasmuch as it asserts or demands the possibility of reciprocity, and therefore of recognition.»* (Bourdieu 1990: 98)

logic of practice is seen as beyond articulation; it is *«supra-reflexive»*. The agent's misrecognition of the logic of practice is attributed, in part, to his rationalization of intent, again relating for Bourdieu, to «time». The agent does not simply act because of an expected future, but also because he is led to where he is by his (and his surrounding's) past (Bourdieu 2012: 79).

The practice of the agent, then, cannot be reduced to his rational and strategic expectations of the outcome of an act (such as he presents it). Practice is only determined by expected future outcomes *in appearance*. The logic of practice, understood as different from theoretical knowledge (Petersen 2004: 150-1), is not to be found *in the results* of practice:

> «*If they seem determined by anticipation of their own consequences, thereby encouraging the finalist illusion, the fact is that, always tending to reproduce the objective structures of which they are the product, they are determined by the past conditions which have produced the principles of their production, that is, by the actual outcome of identical or interchangeable past practices, which coincides with their own outcome to the extent (and only to the extent) that the objective structures of which they are the product are prolonged in the structures within which they function*». (Bourdieu 2012: 72-73)

This quote illustrates the complexity of Bourdieu's agent's liminality between agency and structural influences (on which there is not sufficient space to elaborate): his practice can be seen to be organized as strategies, without being the product of a genuine strategic intention, while at the same time reproducing the objective structures, structuring his practice.

Based on these premises we can outline Bourdieu´s theory of practice. The theory of practice can be described as a theory of *«the mode of generation of practices»* (Bourdieu 2012); that is, a theory of how practices are created rather than how they are played out. For Bourdieu's agent, practice is not the dissemination of meaning or rationality. Rather it is *through* practice that meaning can be created. Thus, it is through the *study of* practice that the researcher can gain access to the layers of meaning connected to what goes on. So, what is it Bourdieu's agents do? They «*(...) construct social reality, individually and also collectively*» (Bourdieu & Waquant 1992: 10). However, Bourdieu's agent is not free in his construction; he has not constructed the categories he puts to work in his work of construction. In other words, Bourdieu's concept of the agent's ability to construct meaning relies on a fundament or a construct already in place for the agent, which the agent cannot control or manipulate, but to which he always must relate. Such constructs, represented by the term «*field*»[4] and the relationship between a field and the habitus (to which we will return), present but also limit options for the agent (Bourdieu 1990: 68). The relationship between field and habitus further contributes to the impossibility of articulating the foundation of one's practice.

The agent's detachment from the principles that structure his action does not imply, however, that the agent does not find meaning in his action, or that his practice can be said to be without meaning. The agent and his actions are more «*to the point*» than what can be recovered through his spontaneous consciousness or the explications he uses (Callewaert 1997). His actions are located within the realm of *ability* rather than *knowledge*, in other words. In this way, the agent's practice is meaningful for him and his surroundings on a practical rather than a logical level. The misrecognition by the agent of the logic of practice (Petersen 1993) can be further explained by the generating principles of habitus (my highlights):

> «(…) *systems of durable, transportable dispositions, structured structures predisposed to function as structuring structures, that is,* **as principles which generate and organize practices** *and representations that can be objectively adapted to their outcomes* **without presupposing a conscious aiming at ends** *or an express mastery of the operations necessary in order to attain them.*» (Bourdieu 1990: 53)

Habitus, as seen by this definition, are dispositions that guide practice without «being used» deliberately by agents (more possessed than in possession of the habitus (Bourdieu 2012: 18)). Habitus can, as such, be understood as providing the agent with tools for practice, or, perhaps more to the point: with potential trajectories. These trajectories are followed *without being read as a map.* Such a lack of deliberation does not imply that practice is not constructed and static, but rather is «*spontaneity without consciousness*» (Bourdieu 1990:56). The trajectories can be altered while underway, to continue our analogy, although one cannot alter the dynamic of the generating principles of the trajectories. Habitus can still enable the agent to act adequately accordingly to

---

4   Described elsewhere as «(…) *a social arena within which struggles or maneuvers take place over specific resources or stakes and access to them (…) Each field, by virtue of its defining content, has a different logic and taken-for-granted structure of necessity and relevance which is both the product and producer of the habitus which is specific and appropriate to the field*» (Jenkins 1992: 84).

the situation: «(...) *the strategy-generating principle enabling agents to cope with unforeseen and ever-changing situations*» (Bourdieu 2012: 72).

Practice is thus neither mechanical nor completely rational. Still, practice has more meaning and function than the agent alludes to. To understand why agents, through practice, «do» more than they «know they do», we must understand habitus as being «(...) *collectively orchestrated without being the product of the organizing action of a conductor*» (Bourdieu 1990: 53). This element of «collectivity» is important for Bourdieu's understanding of habitus and practice, and imperative to my analysis. For our context, this point needs to be highlighted; action and practice are not coincidental, but are understandable and communicable *between* agents, and, at the same time, they are performed collectively without the intention of being collective. The habitus, in Bourdieu's view, helps in making sense of practice, without the agent's attempting to make sense:

> «*The homogeneity of habitus that is observed within the limits of a class of conditions of existence and social conditionings is what causes practices and works to be immediately intelligible and foreseeable, and hence taken for granted. The habitus makes questions of intention superfluous, not only in the production but also in the deciphering of practices and work.*» (Bourdieu 1990: 58)

With this, we see that it is the very mechanism that makes practice meaningful to the agent that simultaneously makes such meaning difficult to reach for the agent. Perhaps paradoxically, practice is simultaneously «*immediately intelligible*» and «*taken for granted*», to use Bourdieu's own words.

In this light, employees in a nursing home unit can be seen as performing their daily tasks as a collective without the conscious choice of a collective performance. Furthermore, the collective practice is taken for granted, it is a «*pre-verbal taking-for-granted of the world that flows from practical sense*» (Bourdieu 1990: 68), in the sense that it not only lacks explicit collective intent but also collective rationalization and collective formulation.

In a perhaps naïve attempt to convey the dynamic of the practical sense of caring staff members in nursing homes - how the practical sense is practiced by them - an analogy of a «pathway» or «trail» can be constructed. When we act, we act based on those who have acted before us and those who act with us, like walking on a trail in the forest. The trail is not particularly distinct nor is it straightforward (as opposed to a road), yet something about our intuition makes us walk it. In an interplay between the body and mind that is almost automatic, we follow the trail, without making explicit deliberations about our choices. We follow the trail without expressing a desire to follow it. Furthermore, the trail is not random or coincidental, people have walked it before, with some kind of purpose or at least meaning; it is there for a reason. Yet the reason is not explicit or even known to us. The trail is most likely a sensible route to where one is going; those who have walked before us did not choose it randomly. One can diverge from the trail, intentionally (if the trail or a part of the trail is clear and easy to see) or unintentionally. Yet something about the landscape surrounding the trail leads us, more often than not, back on the trail. Over time, as we walk it, the trail changes, gradually and perhaps unnoticeably, not necessarily as the result of an intent to change, but because a more sensible path was walked, over time. The trail exists and «works» only because of those who walk it and those who have walked it. Others do/did not create it, being either a divine entity or officials (either God or a representative from the municipality). Such an analogy is far from an adequate depiction of Bourdieu's theoretical framework, or of its applicability to caring staff in our nursing homes, but it does share some common traits. The trail might illustrate that walking is not determined exclusively by explicit intent or by external influence. Nor is the trail walked exclusively based on old habits. Practice is found somewhere in between these influencing bodies. For caring staff in nursing homes the trail is walked, more often than not, *together*; the experienced leading the way, without, in some cases, the explicit intent of doing so.

For Bourdieu, practice is both dynamic and relational, and at the same time, structured. For agents in the nursing home, decisions concerning residents are at the same time based on interactional aspects occurring continuously and on aspects outside the reach of the reflections and negotiations of the agents involved. In this way habitus points to something shared *and at the same time* taken for granted between agents, taking the form of *learned ignorance; «(...) a mode of practical knowledge not comprising knowledge of its principles»* (Bourdieu 2012: 19).

Such is the understanding of the institutional practices in nursing homes: caring staff share taken for granted practice, which makes sense without stating sensibility. Rather than stating the universal applicability of the theory of practice on man, it will suffice for me to state *its particular relevance and transferability to the practices by caring staff in nursing homes* – understood as the institutional practice. A similar argument was raised by Petersen & Callewaert, although on a somewhat larger scale – that of the modern healthcare sector - stating that the pre-conscious orientations steering the practical sense can be considered to be misrecognized *because* of the degree to which procedures are planned in a technocratic and bureaucratic manner (2013: 20).

10.2.2. A fundamental uncertainty and the institutional practice

Before further elaborating on how the theoretical perspectives of the theory of practice can be transferred to our setting, the structuring mechanisms for practice in the nursing homes – the premises of practice - will be revisited. The relationships between practice and structure are not tangible; they are constantly in flux for the practitioner, serendipitous and deceiving for the researcher. Even so, structural mechanisms *work*; they are effective, however different the effect may be.

The structural mechanisms relate to practice in nursing homes differently: both in form and degree of influence. The relationship between the structural mechanisms and practice differs both in time and space; differently within a nursing home or units within a nursing home at different times, and differently between nursing homes. The absence of specific directives and protocols connected to decisions of hospitalization can serve as an example; there are no formal guidelines addressing the issues of hospitalization for caring staff. For the incidents described in the preceding chapters, there were no protocols for those dealing with the situation, no instructions and no textbooks; the «solution» had to be found on the spot. As such, the complex and ambiguous decisions were left to the discretion of the nursing home staff. Thus, variation *can* occur. It does not follow, however, that variation must occur. The structural framework and institutional conditions discussed, facilitate a professional discretion that again facilitates the *possibility of variation*, while the *occurrence of variation* depends, as I have and will argue, on *the institutional practice* at the respective nursing homes.

The uncertainty for caring staff resulting from structural mechanisms is further accentuated by the variation and complexity of the nursing home resident, making continuity vital on several levels. Continuity is, as seen, a prerequisite for understanding the nursing home resident; she is old, frail, dependent and in need of a broad array of assistance and supervision. To make matters more challenging for caring staff, there are many of her, all different, all frail, and all dependent. The skills needed to deal with her, at least to deal with her in a manner by which her varied needs are met, are not easily attainable. They are certainly not passed on to caring staff when entering the nursing home for the first time, nor are they attained through their education. The skills needed to deal with the multitude of residents' challenges, including communication, are not fixed entities one either possesses or not; rather they are inherently ambiguous in the sense of being shifting, varied and non-specific. Caring staff, then, have to acquire skills and practices that have to be interpreted and adjusted continually, both for the neophyte and the experienced.

The uncertainty of the caring staff member is not simply an uncertainty of meeting the unknown, but a *fundamental uncertainty* in the sense of continually operating in an area without ready-made solutions and with shifting premises. This fundamental uncertainty is a premise for the practice of caring staff, in the sense that it is *from where practice is generated*; the fundamental uncertainty *is primal.* Furthermore, the uncertainty is fundamental in the sense that it concerns itself with the most important aspects of their duties: the well-being of the residents, and is, therefore, an uncertainty that must be altered, tamed and made certain. *This process can only be done by the caring staff themselves*, and only *among* the caring staff (rather than being an individual undertaking). Caring staff have no choice but to develop patterns of practice, but, they do not create and implement practice by active deliberation. Such an understanding draws, as we have seen, on Bourdieu's general understanding of a theory of practice, but also, more precisely, on Callewaert's interpretation of it (1997). Callewaert argues, implicitly against frequent adaptations of Bourdieu, that the most pivotal element of the practical sense (for Bourdieu) is not the embodiment of dispositions or the significance of dispositions in general, but rather that the practical sense is *an adequately adapted orientation towards the objective conditions such as they are* (Ibid., Petersen 1993). The practical sense is, in other words, adequate to the area in which they are implemented, more so than perceptions and formulations of adequacy by the agent would imply. The practice of the agent has an accurateness not to be found in spontaneous explanations of it, as the objective condition from which practice is generated is incorporated as an orientation (Callewaert 1997). Such «*principles of orientation*», of which the practical sense can be seen as an actual, everyday implementation, can be presented by the practitioner as governed by rules, but only in the form of rationalizations after the fact (Petersen 1993). *In practice*, the practical sense is accurate, but not theoretical/logical. Furthermore, the agent does not stand alone in such a process, but shares an orientation for practice with those adhering to similar circumstances, thus also sharing an incorporation (Callewaert 1992). The unanimity among agents is not a result of collective calculations or of conscious conformity set against a set of familiar and well known rules, but rather occurs without a form of organized and conscious coordination (Petersen & Callewaert 2013: 122-23). As such, I believe, the institutional practice can be understood: shared, implicit, adequate and relating to the specific conditions at each institution. Following also from this theoretical understanding: practice varies. Practice varies, as it is (implicitly) adapted to the situation and the objective conditions surrounding it: it is strategic without signifying strategy.

To be specific: sets of practices for the caring staff need to be created, constantly re-created and implemented *on-the-spot*, through a *process of learned ignorance* (Callewaert 1997: 13-25, Bourdieu 2012: 19). There are no ready-made, a priori ways of operating as a group of caring staff in the unit, despite the bountiful rules; caring staff are themselves responsible for the creation and implementation of their practice. The precise form and extent of practice, then, is not a given; it needs to be created from the ground up. As such, practice is inherently local, grounded in units or small nursing homes, *because it has to be*. Furthermore, the practice needed is, because of the structuring framework provided and the uncertainty connected to it, inherently and fundamentally *shared, because it has to be*; the institutional practice is *social*.

As such, caring staff in nursing homes develop and implement sets or regimes of practices that can vary between institutions. Although caring staff in nursing homes share the fundamental uncertainty functioning as a premise for the development of the institutional practice, they do not necessarily share the specific traits, forms or «strengths» of the institutional practice. While *the need* to develop patterns of practice can be described as universal for caring staff in nursing homes, the specific forms these patterns take, *how* practice is developed and ultimately plays out, is unique (while internally shared). The forms of practice, in turn, relate to the specific institutional context, in varying and complex ways. Thus, we can identify *the institutional practice* as something local and as more, rather than less, unique, albeit adhering to the same dynamic.

Consequently, nursing homes vary, also, as will be illustrated now, regarding hospitalizations.

10.2.3. Two examples of variation

To a large degree, this dynamic is parallel to that of specific practices of hospitalization. Decisions of hospitalizations are, at least in many instances, embedded within an institutional practice. This can be illustrated through aspects of everyday life in nursing homes which I argue are both parts of an institutional practice *and* of particular importance for decisions of hospitalizations: *knowledge and experience with family, and collaboration with physicians.* These aspects vary greatly between nursing homes, and can therefore explain, at least in part, the variation between them.

> An improvised conversation with a physician in the corridor, Durmstrang. The physician, a consultant working exclusively within geriatric care (as opposed to other physicians at other small nursing homes who only worked part time exclusively with elderly patients), emphasized the importance of knowing the particular and peculiar challenges that are relevant when working in nursing homes: *Especially palliative treatment. We need to be reflective towards palliative treatment, to be serious about it, and I don't think everyone is.* An assisting nurse approached the physician, obviously in a hurry, and told him that they were pressed for time and needed to *get on with it*[5]. About 20 minutes later, while doing his rounds, the physician approached me again, apparently eager to share his thoughts. He continued where he left off: *They*[6] *are also important for it*[7], *and we take that part seriously, I and the institution, that is. But they are also different. To put it in a larger perspective, some, who are «better off» can be more demanding, those who are resourceful demand more from the health sector. They see it as the health sector´s duty to provide all kinds of support and treatment, including extensive treatment in the nursing home as opposed to palliative treatment. Others do not see it that way.*

As seen, communicating with family members of residents, both on admission and later, is important for when severe or acute illness occurs and for the general preparation for such incidents. In a majority of the qualitative studies

---

5   Referring to the visitation of residents.
6   Referring to family members.
7   Referring to palliative treatment.

described, *«pressure from family»* is highlighted as highly influential for hospitalizations of nursing home residents (Arendts & Howard 2010, Bottrell et al. 2001, Hutt et al. 2011, Jablonski et al. 2007, Kayser-Jones et al. 1989, Lamb et al. 2011, Lopez 2009, Phillips et al. 2006, Shanley et al. 2011). It is argued that families of residents pressure caring staff, physicians and residents, to hospitalize residents, on many occasions contrary to the recommendations of staff and/or the (at times presumed) wishes of residents. Pressure from family, it would seem, is omnipresent in nursing homes, including Norwegian ones (Dreyer et al. 2010, Hov et al. 2009) and is influential for the practices of staff. But how does pressure from family factor in in explaining *variation*? Pressure from family, I will argue, depends on the approaches and familiarity between caring staff/physician/unit leadership and family, especially connected to preparing for decisions to come, regarding potential hospitalizations and/or end of life care. Nursing homes within our sample vary considerably in such approaches, leading to different levels of familiarity with and knowledge about family members, and, ultimately, different degrees of pressure when illness occurs. As such, *how* staff in nursing homes and units relate to family members, concretely and in general, and their familiarity with each other can influence specific decisions on hospitalizations.

This particular nursing home in the included excerpt above for instance, had a more explicit and systematized approach towards involving family members in discussions about treatment and palliative care, on admission and later. Consequentially, the nursing home was better equipped to deal with pressure from family, even from what could be considered demanding family members, than other nursing homes. As illustrated by this nursing home, continuity in relationships in the form of familiarity between the respective agents, can breed *further continuity* in relationships, and vice versa. For nursing homes where interaction with family members is not routinized to such an extent as in the above example, familiarity with family members can be difficult to attain and/or establish when needed, potentially leading to assertive and sudden pressure when a decision-process occurs.

Relatedly, physicians' involvement with family vary considerably within our sample. Some have virtually no contact, some have formalized contact in the form of meetings with next of kin on the resident's arrival at the nursing home, while some have extensive and continual contact. Consequently, the *content* of the communication between physicians and family members varies significantly.

Some, but far from all, address the issue of potential hospitalizations, either when residents move in and/or in the beginning stages of an illness. While some physicians leave these tasks to caring staff, many caring staff see the advantages of physicians handling such a delicate matter, in part, because *they immediately get more respect*, as one registered nurse put it.

Similarly to the few research articles addressing the issue (Dreyer et al. 2010, McGregor et al. 2010), physicians at the included nursing homes who had experience with and knowledge of residents and families were better positioned to discuss issues relating to end of life. At Durmstrang, for example, the physician addressed the issue of potential hospitalizations with families and residents on resident admission. At other nursing homes, a physician addressed the issues at a later stage, or not at all, leaving the issue to the discretion of caring staff.

Different forms of physician employment lead to different forms of integration and collaboration between physicians and caring staff, and between physicians, caring staff and family. Continuity of physicians, in the form of size of position and tenure at the nursing home (in part also general experience with elderly patients), is influential for how well equipped physicians are at evaluating, understanding and treating nursing home residents, in other words. Continuity of physicians relates not solely to technical knowledge, but also to how integrated they are within the institutional practice. This influence also works in reverse: the physician with experience and knowledge of the unit and the residents in it, will influence the respective institutional practices, as will be elaborated on shortly. In general, physicians vary, within and outside our sample, significantly in experience and knowledge of the units. *Continuity of physicians, therefore, can be an extremely important factor in understanding and explaining variation in the practice of hospitalization.*

> My first meeting with the only physician at a small nursing home (name withheld) led to a short conversation leaving a lasting impression. The physician, employed through the municipality and performing his duty-work one day a week at the nursing home, expressed, after getting a brief overview of my project, a grave dissatisfaction with the working conditions. He conveyed a feeling of being pressured, that there was too much to do in too little time (which he explained frantically, as he needed to hurry on): *This, what I do here, really is irresponsible. There simply isn´t enough time. I really wish I didn´t do this, because I feel responsible for something I cannot control.*

10.2.4. Variation in hospitalization and the institutional practice

Physician collaboration and family interaction can explain variation in practices (and rates) of hospitalization. These aspects are also components of the institutional practice; how caring staff (or caring staff and physician) interact with family is – in effect – not part of the formalized set of guidelines or even routines; they are rather part of the implicit, taken for granted practices, shared among practitioners locally. Caring staff act towards family as they do as a part of their practical sense.

The differences between nursing homes regarding these (and other) aspects of everyday practices in nursing homes can also be found between units within the same nursing home. Two units at Acre Woods will be revisited.

In *the unit*, a form of collective positioning towards non-hospitalization was prevalent in accounts of «the collective identity of the unit» and, in my opinion, in approaches, sentiments and actions beyond those which were articulated. The positioning was expressed as being strongly connected to the collaboration with their physician, in contrast to other units (including *the other unit*), and their respective collaboration with their physicians.

> *When it comes to how we deal with hospitals, for instance, well, I don´t know quite how to put it, but we can sense a different attitude in other physicians than ours. So sometimes we are hesitant to call another physician, because he will probably hospitalize more, compared to our unit. Sometimes it is better to wait until our physician is available, or call him late at night. This might not be the correct procedure, but I feel that it is right, and have to be honest about that.* (Caring staff member, *the unit*)

The excerpt, alludes to the understanding of caring staff (and physician) in *the unit* of their positioning towards hospitalizations; they would prefer not to hospitalize, if given a choice. Such a preference is presented as being founded in altruistic motives: giving the old and frail resident comfort, familiarity and peace, trumping that of treatment, medicine and life extension. Furthermore, the residents, it is assumed, would prefer to stay in the unit. Such a position is taken while relating to other units in the nursing home and is, simultaneously, firmly rooted in a notion of *practice* towards what we do (as opposed to what others do).

How this particular unit, the main unit of fieldwork, is presented as being different with regard to positioning towards hospitalizations, is connected not only to other units at the nursing home or other nursing homes, but also specifically to one other unit in the nursing home. This *other unit* is especially effective for the process of mirroring *the unit*, in part because it employs another physician. And this *other unit* is seen as positioned differently towards hospitalization and treatment, relating to its relationship with their physician; they will give their residents more aggressive regimens of treatment and hospitalize more frequently.

At the *other unit*, positioning towards hospitalization or in-house care was not expressed as explicitly as within *the unit*. When doing so, the emphasis was on either treating in-house or abstaining from treatment at all. Two differences from *the unit*, then, can be found: the collective positioning towards hospitalization/treatment/non-treatment is not as distinct or encompassing as for *the unit*, and when expressed, hospitalizations and in-house treatment (as opposed to non-treatment) were presented as valid options, to a higher degree than for *the unit*.

The differences, more often than not in the form of nuances and degrees, were conveyed collectively at report meetings, during physician visitations, and during interviews with unit leadership. The unit leader of *the other unit* did, for example, voice a sentiment towards avoiding hospitalizations, if possible, but did so based on a wish to *treat residents in the unit*, rather than based on a preference of avoiding medical treatment altogether. In *the unit*, meanwhile, similar sentiments were expressed, but *non-treatment*, as opposed to *in-house treatment*, was emphasized as an alternative to hospitalization. The difference between the two units illustrates a general point relevant for all nursing homes; the «choice» institutions have to make cannot be reduced to (as it is in a majority of the research literature) a choice between hospitalization and non-treatment (palliative care, for instance), but rather between hospitalization, non-treatment and/or in-house treatment. Nursing homes and/or units can have a proclivity towards one of these preferences, or two. *The unit* for instance, had a proclivity towards in-house treatment and non-treatment, while *the other unit* had a proclivity towards in-house treatment and hospitalization.

The unit is, as such, presented by caring staff as different from *the other unit* regarding treatment, end-of-life care and hospitalization. However, the differences between the units relate to more than rhetoric; they are visible also in everyday life in the units, for instance at report meetings and during physician visits.

Collaboration with the physician in *the unit*

The weekly meeting between unit leadership and the physician takes place in the office of the unit leader. The unit leader, another registered nurse and the physician are present. After some initial conversation and small talk, they prepare for the weekly review of residents: the registered nurse by reading from journals/charts in paper form, the physician by placing himself in front of the computer to get access to the electronic journals if needed, while the unit leader sits behind her desk. The registered nurse is «running the show»: she initiates the topics of conversation and presents the residents one by one, sometimes informing the others, sometimes asking questions. The physician and the unit leader occasionally respond to the presentation of the registered nurse, sometimes adding a detail to the presentation, sometimes answering a question. All three demonstrate detailed knowledge of the residents, their current state and their regimens of medicine. In general, the tone is informal and relaxed: they seem comfortable with each other and appear to value the insight and opinions of one another. On several occasions, the registered nurse would correct the physician, regarding the day of an event for instance, to which the physician would smile and thank the registered nurse. They alter between discussing the general condition of residents and their specific regimens of medicine, both in terms of developments in the last week. The registered nurse informs the others of significant changes in general health for four of the residents, warranting an increase or decrease in medical treatment. Together they discuss how the residents in question should be approached, both in terms of their «psychosocial» and medical well-being. An increase in or an excessive use of medication is stressed several times as unwanted. Such an emphasis was, to my understanding, primarily implicit among the three: they attempted to find other solutions than medical treatment when they could (without stating the need to), and resorted to medical treatment when they deemed they had to. One resident, who suffered from back pain after a recent fall, was given an increase in current medication, after a rather long deliberation, while another resident, gradually becoming more tired in recent weeks according to the registered nurse, was taken off her medication. Together they decided that increased attention towards activities and movement was the right path for the resident, while monitoring possible changes in restlessness and «wandering».

Collaboration with the physician in *the other unit*

The weekly meeting between unit leadership and the physician takes place in the office of the unit leader. The assisting unit leader (in the absence of the unit leader) is alone with the physician, while another registered nurse joins them towards the end. More familiar with the collaboration and atmosphere between the physician and caring staff in *the unit*, I found this meeting to be considerably different from the very onset. The physician was clearly in charge: in the way he was seated (in the center of the room), in the use of supplies (having control both over the paper and electronic journal system) and by being in charge of presentations and discussions. The physician presented one resident at a time, spending considerable time on residents particularly regarding their respective regimens of medicine. Occasionally he would confer with the assisting nurse, more often than not to get confirmation of his own opinions. The assisting nurse did not interrupt the presentation of the physician, nor otherwise oppose him. The medical well-being of residents was almost exclusively in focus: the medication of residents was changed or slightly adjusted for approximately half of the residents. While registering the changes, the physician would talk about the qualities and effects of the various forms of medication (perhaps for my benefit), demonstrating also a great and detailed knowledge of all residents, and their recent development. The assisting unit leader, meanwhile, would take on the role of an observer.

During physician visits in *the other unit*, attention was directed at the medical treatment of residents, not in opposition to *the unit*, but to a higher degree than for *the unit*. While this was also done in *the unit*, problematizing the benefits of rigorous treatment (in some cases also problematizing whether one should treat at all) seemed to be an integral part of the routine of visitations in *the unit* and less prevalent in *the other unit*. The biggest difference still seemed to be that which is not explicitly addressed. In *the unit*, a silent consensus between physician and unit leadership (as between unit leadership and the rest of the caring staff at other times) seemed to be in effect when discussing what were considered «difficult cases». Everything did not need to be said; the reasons for downscaling medicine for a dying resident, for instance, was agreed upon, but not explicitly discussed in detail. Nor was what can be considered a general approach towards non-medical treatment of residents discussed explicitly: it was more of a premise for what was to be discussed.

As such, the positioning of caring staff in *the unit* is not only a question of identity construction (relating to the need for a sense of community discussed previously), but also, and perhaps primarily, a dissemination of differences *in practice*. Caring staff in *the unit* act in a certain manner towards hospitalization, different *in form and degree* from how *the other unit* act towards hospitalization.

In conclusion, two particularly important features of the broader concepts of continuity – family and physician interaction - can simultaneously illustrate how an institutional practice affects the everyday life of nursing homes and how it can generate variation for specific decisions of hospitalizations. Even though caring staff in nursing homes share a fundamental uncertainty that functions as a premise for an institutional practice, they do not share the specific traits or forms of it. The need to develop regimes of practice are universal for caring staff, while the specific forms these take are unique and shared locally. The result is different practices of hospitalization between nursing homes and even units within a nursing home.

10.3. Concluding remarks: solutions?

Following the argumentation, practices of hospitalizations are, as an integrated part of the institutional practice, a) shared, b) local and c) discretionary. Furthermore, practices of hospitalizations can vary between (and sometimes within) institutions. That is not to say that practices of hospitalizations are coincidental, or that the development of sets of practices of hospitalizations appears from a vacuum, independently from the micro and macro context of the nursing homes. Rather, I will argue that sets of practices of hospitalizations are conditional, in the sense that they do relate to a wide range of structural mechanisms, of various importance in time and space, and generally non-determinant in effect. The analysis has shown that we do need to look at each individual nursing home, in depth, and not simply at their formal characteristics. By the sheer virtue of being nursing homes, the institutions are inexplicably influenced by a structural framework and institutional conditions to which they must adhere. These structuring mechanisms do not, however, *determine* practice: a set of conditions will not necessarily lead to a set of practices. Nor is the relationship between the structural mechanisms and practice absolute or universal, in the sense that nursing homes with similar conditions necessarily develop similar sets of practices. Rather, practices of hospitalization differ because it is part of the institutional practice, *which by its very nature and formative process must vary*, depending particularly on continuity. Variation, therefore, is invariable and (as opposed to the view of the majority of research) unavoidable. No variation in practices of hospitalization would, contrarily, be an inexplicable coincidence.

Where does this conclusion leave us? First and foremost, generalizations of nursing homes' practices based on formal characteristics must be avoided. There is no typical nursing home with high rates of hospitalization, or a typical nursing home with low rates, at least within the sample of nursing homes in this study. In other words, and returning to the sample, there are no defining characteristics shared within the two respective samples that would explain why they hospitalize more or less than the average nursing home; there is no clear and obvious connection between shared characteristics of the two respective samples and our defined outcome, rates of hospitalization.

As such, we cannot isolate what makes a nursing home hospitalize more or less than others, *as universally valid rules.*

Again: where does that leave us? Can we, instead, isolate traits or qualities of nursing homes more ideal for practices of hospitalization than others? I believe we can speak, at least, of *significance* of traits and qualities.

Continuity, as an *aspect* of several discussed factors, as opposed to their particular qualities (small/large nursing home, direct/indirect employment of physician, coverage of the respective professional groups), seems to be of great significance and has been shown to be directly influential for practices, including that of hospitalizations. Knowledge of specific residents, experience in the unit and familiarity between caring staff and resident can all contribute to preventing and avoiding injuries or ailments that could, potentially, lead to hospitalizations. Continuity then, can in some instances prevent the decision-making process altogether. In other instances, continuity can be an instrument in the decision-making process, to the benefit of staff and residents.

Continuity, I believe, is a prerequisite for dealing more or less soundly with ambiguous decisions that are typical for instances where hospitalizations are considered. Continuity, then, in its many forms, can be seen as an ideal, often underappreciated by decision-makers and researchers alike. The significance of continuity should not, though, be understood simply as dependent on length of tenure, but rather as connected to the stability of staff/resident interaction on several interrelated levels. Staff should know (and should be allowed to know) their residents, while residents should have familiar and knowledgeable staff members tending to them.

As for traits of nursing homes, isolating «correct» practices of hospitalizations are problematic. As previously discussed, high (or low) rates of hospitalization, *in themselves* should not be considered unwarranted. Nor should variation in hospitalization, *it itself*, be seen as «unnatural». Several aspects of continuity, meanwhile, have been shown to contribute to explaining variation between institutions; stability in caring staff/physician relationships, for instance, can lead to a certain practice of hospitalization. Still, I will argue that continuity does not necessarily lead either to higher or lower rates of hospitalization, but rather that decisions *can be more adequately and soundly founded* based on continuity of caring staff. Perhaps rather than fixating on «correct rates of hospitalizations», researchers and practitioners could benefit from directing attention towards providing sound environments in which decisions are made; decisions on hospitalizations can be more or less soundly founded, both when leading to a hospitalization, and not. Decisions can also be poorly founded, both when residents are hospitalized, and not. As such, *a rate of hospitalization*, in itself, should not be considered an indicator of quality, especially not on an institutional level. That is not to say that policy makers and researchers alike cannot strive for increasing quality related to transfers of residents from nursing homes, but should, rather, direct attention towards what can lead to an ideal understanding of nursing home residents, rather than the quantities of transfers.

10.4. Meeting a resident: understanding Alice

Alice

Alice was never one to make a huge impression on those around her. Her small physical frame and the fact that she would usually sit in a faraway corner of the large common room, almost as if hiding, mirrored that of her presence in the unit in general. She did not interact much with other residents, she did not ask much of the staff - she did not make much of a fuss. Alice has lost most of her hearing, some of her sight, and is generally physically frail, hardly able to walk on her own. However, she appears to have a clear mind, giving coherent responses when asked, although seldom raising issues herself. My impression of her is of someone who struggles with her loss of hearing, leading both to anxiety and modesty, further reinforcing an already introvert demeanor. The staff, in my opinion, seemed to have developed a liking for her, but at the same time did not spend a lot of time with her, perhaps because they could afford not to, perhaps they felt Alice did not want them to. For the caring staff, Alice was «easy to care for», both in the sense of not needing or demanding much care and attention and in the sense of being «easy to read»; the caring staff seemed to have figured out what and when Alice needed assistance. When seen or heard outside her seat in the common room, Alice was usually on her way to or from the toilet, either alone, cautiously walking with her walking frame, or together with a staff member.

I too did not spend much time with Alice; she seemed to blend in with her surroundings while my attention was drawn towards other, more «visible» residents. In the latter part of my fieldwork, I wanted to remedy my lack of attention towards her. I had talked to her before, or rather exchanged pleasantries that seldom developed into more. When approaching Alice, I, as I have seen some of the caring staff do, crouched down close to her, to get onto her «level». Talking loudly, a conversation of sort transpired. Her story, mostly a monologue as a consequence of lack of hearing, was a sad one: she said that she realized she was getting old, and did not have much time left. Still, she said, she was glad for each day. Her biggest regret was not having a close relationship with her family. Alice said with a slight tremor in her voice: *They almost never come to visit.* Alice's´ attention seemed to drift away after this.

The next time I approached Alice, shortly after the above conversation, she was noticeably more welcoming towards me. She smiled on my approach, and, as opposed to before, took the initiative of starting a conversation: *I´m ok, a bit tired, only,* she said after greeting me. *But my senses are getting worse and worse, so I´m tired all the time. I hope I don´t have much time left now.* A small pause before continuing: *Well, that´s how it is to grow old, I suppose. I´ve lived for a long time, almost 100 years. Imagine that!* She pauses again, seemingly lost in thought, while I simply nod in response: *And it´s just so quiet here. It is difficult to contact people* (she looks around the room). *But it is good that you people come here and check that everything is going as it should* (referring, to my surprise, to my role as a researcher, which I was not sure had been properly conveyed to her). *I get what I want and need here. Good food and a lot of it. I have even gained several kilos since coming here!* Alice laughs, a rare sound in the unit, while an assisting nurse starts preparing the table for dinner, signaling the end of our discussion.

During the next couple of weeks, I got the impression of Alice becoming increasingly uneasy. She did not seem at ease when seated, as she usually did, and, perhaps more strikingly, rose and walked aimlessly around many times every day, obviously discomforted. Her walks to the toilet, though frequent before, became an hourly event, to the point of being viewed by some staff members as compulsive. These frequently and sudden walks to the toilet became a concern for many caring staff members, as they were afraid that Alice would fall. As discussed in several report meetings, the caring staff paid close attention to Alice in this period, at least when they could.

One evening in particular displayed Alice´s growing anxiety and the staff's attempts to calm her. Alice said that she expected a visitor later that evening, before continuing, visibly stressed and shaken up: *But I don´t know if she will show or not. It´s my daughter, you see. We are very close, from before. And I don´t know when she will come.* Alice looked around the room as if looking for her visitor. A relatively new assisting nurse entered the common room and, after hearing Alice's concerns, approached her: *On Friday, Alice, she will come on Friday. Today is Thursday.* The assisting nurse left shortly thereafter, onto other tasks. Alice did not seem to apprehend the message and continued to voice her prior concern. About five minutes later the assisting nurse returned and was called upon by Alice. Alice asked if she could call her daughter to ask again when she would come. The assisting nurse replied that she would have to wait until her daughter finished her shift at her job. When saying this, Alice, untypically, grabbed the assisting nurse's wrist, held it tight, as if pleading for assistance. The assisting nurse explained about the daughter's job while trying to distance herself physically from Alice. Unable to do so because of Alice's grip, she used her free hand to loosen the grip and walked away and out of the common room. Alice was not put at ease. About five minutes later, she rose up and headed for the corridor. I talked to her, and attempted to stop her by repeating the message of the assisting nurse. She returned to her seat but still she did not settle. For about 10 minutes, she asked the same question: *Do you think she is coming?* whilst occasionally standing up and walking a couple of paces before settling down again. Another, more experienced assisting nurse, who apparently had been informed of Alice's state by others, entered the common room. She, in a much calmer tone and taking more time compared to the other assisting nurse, explained the situation to Alice. She did not add anything, but explained it slower, in a clearer voice, repeated a couple of points, all the while holding Alice's hand and stroking it. Alice´s reaction was visibly different from before: she laughed loudly, hit her hands on her thighs in enjoyment and said: *Thank you, thank you, and thank you!*

Two days later, Alice´s mood and behavior were still uneasy, still displaying apparent anxiety. After seeing her like this and talking to her, struck by the remarkable similarity to two days before, I asked the assisting nurse who had calmed Alice, what had happened regarding the visit. She explained, while not concealing her displeasure, that the daughter had not arrived at all. Alice had *been like that* for the entirety of the two preceding days, *poor thing*, the assisting nurse added. Meanwhile, I overheard Alice asking a registered nurse if she could call her daughter, to which it was replied that now was not a good time. Later, during a short break in the nurses' station, I asked the registered nurse for her take on the situation. She explained that an assisting nurse had in fact called the daughter last night, and had been chided for asking about visitation, as the daughter had taken the call as unwanted pressure from the staff to get her to visit more often. The registered nurse shrugged her shoulders, as if frustrated by a situation with no possible ideal outcome.

Source of data

Ackermann, R.J. 2001. Nursing home practice: Strategies to manage most acute and chronic illness without hospitalization. *Geriatrics 5* Vol. 56: 37-48.

Anderson, R.A., Hsieh, P., & Su, H. 1998. Resource allocation and resident outcomes in nursing homes: Comparisons between the best and worst. *Research in Nursing & Health* 21: 297-313.

Anderson, R.A., Issel, L.M., & McDaniel, R.R. 2003. Nursing homes as complex adaptive systems: relationship between management practice and resident outcomes. *Nursing Research 52*(1): 12-21

Anphalahan, M. & Gibson, S.J. 2008. Geriatric syndromes as predictors of adverse outcomes of hospitalization. *Internal Medicine Journal* Vol. 38: 16-21.

Arendts, G. & Howard, K. 2010. The interface between residential aged care and the emergency department: a systematic review. *Age and Ageing* 39: 306-312.

Arendts, G., Quine, S. & Howard, K. 2013, Decision to transfer to an emergency department from residential aged care: a systematic review of qualitative research. *Geriatrics & Gerontology International 13*(4): 825-833.

Armstrong, P., Banerjee, A., Szebehely, M., Armstrong, H., Daly, T. & Lafrance, S. 2009. *They Deserve Better: The Long-term Care Experience in Canada and Scandinavia.* Canadian Centre for Policy Alternatives. Canada.

Armstrong, P. 2013. Puzzling skills: feminist political economy approaches. *CRS/RCS,* 50.3. 2013: 256-283

Banaaszak-Holl, J. & Hines, M.A. 1996. Factors associated with nursing home staff turnover. *The Gerentologist* 4, Vol. 36: 512-517.

Barker, W.H., Zimmer, J.G., Hall, W.J., Ruff, B.C., Freundlich, C.B., & Eggert, G.M. 1994. Rates, patterns, causes, and costs of hospitalization of nursing home residents: A population based study. *Am J Public Health* 1994; 84(10):1615.

Bjelland, A.K. 1982. *Aldring og Identitetskrise.* Bergen Studies in Social Anthropology no 27, University of Bergen

Boockvar, K., Gruber-Baldini, A., Burton, L, Zimmerman, S., May, C. & Magaziner, J. 2005. Outcomes of infection in nursing home residents with and without early hospital transfer. *Journal of the American Geriatrics Society* 53: 590-596.

Bottrell, M.M., O'Sullivan, F.J., Robbins, M.A., Mitty, E.L., & Mezey, M.D. 2001. Transferring dying nursing home residents to the hospital: DON perspectives on the nurse's role in transfer decisions. *Geriatric Nursing and Home Care 22*(6): 313-317.

Bourdieu, P. 1990. *The Logic of Practice.* Polity Press, Cambridge.

Bourdieu, P. 1999a. *The Weight of the World.* Oxford Polity.

Bourdieu, P. 1999b. *Meditasjoner.* Oslo: Pax.

Bourdieu, P. 2003. Participant objectivation. *The Journal of the Royal Anthropological Institute 9*(2): 281-294

Bourdieu, P. 2012 [1977]. *Outline of a Theory of Practice.* Cambridge University Press. Cambridge.

Bourdieu, P., Chamboredon, J.C., & Passeron, J.C. 1991. *The Craft of Sociology: Epistemological Preliminaries.* Walter de Gruyter. Berlin – New York.

Bourdieu, P. & Wacquant, L.J.D. 1992. *An Invitation to Reflexive Sociology.* Polity Press. Cambridge.

Brooks, S., Warshaw, G., Hasse, L. & Kues, J.R. 1994. The physician decision-making process in transferring nursing home patients in the hospital. *Arch Intern Med 1994*: 154: 902-908.

Callewaert, S. 1992. *Kultur, Pædagogik og Videnskab, Om Pierre Bourdieus habitusbegrep og praktikteori.* Viborg: Akademisk Forlag A/S.

Callewaert, S. 1997. *Bourdieu-studier*, Institutt for Filosofi, Pædagogok og retorikk, Københavns Universitet.

Carter, M.W. 2003a. Variations in hospitalization rates among nursing home residents: the role of discretionary hospitalization. *Health Services Research 4*, Vol. 38, pp: 1177-1206.

Carter, M.W. 2003b. Factors associated with ambulatory care-sensitive hospitalizations among nursing home residents. *Journal of Aging Health* 15: 295.

Carter, M.W. & Porell, F.W. 2003. Variations in hospitalization rates among nursing home residents: the role of facility and market attributes. *The Gerontologist* 2003: 43(2): 175-191.

Carter, M.W., & Porell, F.W. 2005. Vulnerable populations at risk of potentially avoidable hospitalizations: The case of nursing home residents with Alzheimer's disease. *American Journal of Alzheimer's Disease and Other Dementias,* 20: 349-358.

Carusone, S.C., Loeb, M. & Lohfeld, L. 2006a. A clinical pathway for treating pneumonia in the NH: part I: the nursing perspective. *Journal of the American Medical Directors Association 7*(5): 271-278.

Carusone, S.C., Loeb, M. & Lohfeld, L. 2006b. A clinical pathway for treating pneumonia in the NH: part II: the administrators' perspective and how it differs from nurses' views. *Journal of the American Medical Directors Association 7*(5): 279-286.

Castle, N.G. 2001a. Administrator turnover and quality of care in nursing homes. *The Gerontologist 41*(6): 757-767

Castle, N.G. 2001b. Relocation of the elderly. *Medical Care Research and Review 2001*; 58: 291-333.

Castle, N.G. 2005. Turnover begets turnover. *The Gerontologist 45*(2): 186-195.

Castle, N. & Mor, V. 1996. Hospitalization of nursing home residents: a review of the literature, 1980-1995. *MCR&R 2*, Vol.53: 123-148.

Castle, N.G., Engberg, J. & Anderson, R.A. 2007. Job satisfaction of nursing home administrators and turnover. *Medical Care Research and Review. Vol. 64. Nr. 2*: 191-211.

Cheng, H.Y., Tonorezos, E., Zorowitz, R., Novotny, J., Dubin, S., & Maurer, M.S. 2006. Inpatient care for nursing home patients: an opportunity to improve transitional care. *Journal of American Medical Directors Association* 2006: 7(6): 383-387.

Cohen-Mansfield, J. & Lipson, S., Horton, D. 2003a. Which signs and symptoms warrant involvement of medical staff? The definition and identification of status-change events in the nursing home. *Behavioral Medicine* Vol. 29: 115-120.

Cohen-Mansfield, J. & Lipson, S. Horton, D. 2003b. Medical decision-making process in the nursing home: a comparison of physician and nurse perspectives. *Journal of Gerontologigal nursing* 32: 14-21.

Cohen-Mansfield, J. & Lipson, S. 2006. To hospitalize or not to hospitalize? That is the question: an analysis of decision making in the nursing home. *Behavioral Medicine 2,* Vol. 32: 64-70.

Coleman, E.A. 2003. Falling through the cracks: Challenges and opportunities for improving transitional care for persons with continuous complex care needs. *Journal American Ger Society* 2003(51): 549-555.

Coleman, E.A. & Berenson, R.A. 2004. Lost in transition: Challenges and opportunities for improving the quality of transitional care. *Annals of Internal Medicine 2004*: 140: 533-536.

Collier, E., & Harrington, C. 2008. Staffing characteristics, turnover rates, and quality of resident care in nursing facilities. *Research in Gerontological Nursing.* Vol 1, No 3: 157-169.

Creditor, M.C. 1993. Hazards of hospitalization of the elderly. *Annals of Internal Medicine 3,* Vol. 118: 219-223.

Culler, S.D., Parchman, M.L., & Przybylski, M. 1998. Factors related to potentially preventable hospitalizations among the elderly. *Med Care* 36: 804-817.

Cwinn, M.A., Forster, A.J., Cwinn, A.A., Hebert, G., Calder, L. & Stiell, I.G. 2009. Prevalence of information gaps for seniors transferred from nursing homes to the emergency department. *Canadian Journal of Emergency Medicine*, vol. 11, no. 5: 462-472.

Davies, C. 1995. Competence versus care? Gender and caring work revisited. *Acta Sociologica, 38*(1), 17-31.

Decker, F.H. 2006. Nursing staffing and the outcomes of nursing home stays. *Medical Care* 44: 812-821.

Decker, F.H. 2008. The relationship of nursing staff to the hospitalization of nursing home residents. *Research in Nursing & Health* Vol. 31: 238-251.

Dellefield, M.E. 2000. Staffing in nursing homes and quality indicators. *Journal of Gerontological Nursing 26*(6): 14-28.

Dosa, D. 2005. Should I hospitalize my resident with nursing home-acquired pneumonia? *JAMDA,* 2005 Sep-Oct 6(5): 327-333.

Dreyer, A., Forde, R. & Nortvedt, P. 2010 Life-prolonging treatment in NHs: how do physicians and nurses describe and justify their own practice? *Journal of Medical Ethics* 36(7): 396-400.

Esping-Andersen, G. 1990. *The Three Worlds of Welfare Capitalism,* Cambridge, Polity Press.

Fjær, E.G. & Vabø, M. 2013. Shaping social situations: A hidden aspect of care work in nursing homes. *Journal of Aging Studies* 27: 419-427.

Flacker, J.M., Won, A., Kiely, D.K. & Iloputaife, I. 2001. Differing perceptions of end-of-life care in long-term care. *Journal of Palliative Medicine* 4: 9-13.

Førde, R., Pedersen, R., Nordtvedt, P., Aasland, O.G. 2006. Får eldreomsorgen nok ressurser? *Tidsskrift for Den norske legeforening* 126: 1913-1916.

Freiman, M.P., & Murtaugh, C.M. 1993. The determinants of the hospitalization of nursing home residents. *Journal of Health Economics* 11: 349-359.

Fried, T. & Mor, V. 1997. Frailty and hospitalization of long-term nursing home residents. *Journal of the American Geriatrics Society 45* (3): 265-269.

Gautun, H. & Hermansen, Å. 2011. *Eldreomsorgen under press: Kommunenes helse – og omsorgstilbud til eldre.* Fafo-rapport 2011: 12.

Godden, S. & Pollock, A.M. 2001. The use of acute hospital services by elderly residents of nursing and residential care homes. *Health Soc Care Commy 9*(6): 367-374.

Goffman, E. 1959. *The Presentation of Self in Everyday Life.* Doubleday Anchor Books. New York.

Goffman, E. 1961. *Asylums: Essays on the Social Situation of Mental Patients and other Inmates.* Anchor Books. New York.

Goffman, Erving. 1971 [2010]. *Relations in Public: Microstudies of the Public Order.* Transaction Publishers. New Brunswick (U.S.A) & London (U.K.).

Grabowski, D.C., Stewart, K.A., Broderick, S.M. & Coots, L.A. 2008. Predictors of nursing home hospitalization: a review of the literature. *Medical Care Research and Review 3,* Vol. 65: 3-39.

Graverholt, B., Riise, T., Jamvedt, G., Ranhoff, A.H., Krüger, K. & Nortvedt, M.W. 2011. Acute hospital admissions among nursing home residents: a population-based observational study. *Health Services Research* 11: 126.

Graverholt, B., Riise, T., Jamvedt, G., Husebø. B.S. & Nortvedt, M.W. 2013. Acute hospital admissions from nursing homes: predictors of unwarranted variation? *Scandinavian Journal of Public Health. 41*(4): 359-365.

Gruneir, A., Miller, S.C., Intrator, O. & Mor, V. 2007. Hospitalization of nursing home residents with cognitive impairments: The influence of organizational features and state policies. *Gerontologist* 4

Hampson, I. & Junor, A. 2010. Putting the process back in. Rethinking service sector skills. *Work, Employment & Society 24*(3): 526-545.

Harnett, T., Jönson, H., & Wästerfors, D. 2012. *Makt och Vanmakt på äldreboende.* Studentlitteratur AB. Lund.

Harrington, C., Zimmerman, D., Karon, S.L., Robinson, J. & Beutel, P. 2000. Nursing home staffing and its relationship to deficiencies. *Journal of Gerontology: Social Sciences*: 55B: 278-287.

Harrington, C., Choiniere, J., Goldman, M., Jacosen, F.F., Lloyd, L., McGregor, M., Stamatopolos, V. & Szebehely, M. 2012. Nursing home staffing standards and staffing levels in six countries. *Journal of Nursing Scholarship 44*(1): 88-98.

Hauge, S. 2004. *Jo mere vi er sammen, jo gladere vi blir? – ein feltmetodologisk studie av sjukeheimen som heim.* Doctoral dissertation. Oslo: University of Oslo, Faculty of Medicine.

Hofacker, S.V, Naalsund, P., Iversen, G.S., & Rosland, J.H. 2010. Akutte innleggelser fra sykehjem til sykehus i livets sluttfase. *Tidsskrift for Den norske legeforening* Nr. 17: 130: 1721-1724.

Holmeide, A. & Eimot, M. 2010. *Bemanning i kommunal helse- og omsorgstjeneste.* Oslo: Analysesenteret.

Horn, S.D., Buerhaus, P., Bergstrom, N. & Smout, R.J. 2005. RN staffing time and outcomes of long-stay nursing home residents. *AJN 11,* Vol. 105: 58-70.

Hov, R., Athlin, E. & Hedelin, B. 2009. Being a nurse in NH for patients on the edge of life. *Scandinavian Journal of Caring Sciences* 23: 651-659.

Hujala, A., & Rissanen, S. 2011. Organization aesthetics in nursing homes. *Journal of Nursing Management 19*(4): 439-448

Husebø, B.S. & Husebø, S. 2004. Etiske avgjørelser ved livets slutt i sykehjem. *Tidsskrift for Den norske legeforening* 124: 2926-2927

Husebø, B.S. & Husebø, S. 2005. Sykehjemmene som arena for terminal omsorg – hvordan gjør vi det i praksis? *Tidsskrift for Den Norske legeforening;* 125: 1352-1354.

Hutt, E., Ecord, M., Eilertsen, T.B., Fredrickson, E., & Kramer, A.M. 2002. Precipitants of emergency room visits and acute hospitalization in short-stay medicare nursing home residents. *Journal of the American Geriatrics Society 50*: 223-229.

Hutt, E., Ruscin, J.M., Linnebur, S.A., Fish, D.N., Oman, K.S., Fink, R.M., Radcliff, T.A., Van Dorsten, B., Liebrecht, D., Fish, R. & McNulty, M.C. 2011. A multifaceted intervention to implement guidelines did not affect hospitalization rates for NH-acquired pneumonia. *Journal of the American Medical Directors Association 12*(7): 499-507.

Ingstad, K. 2010. Arbeidsforhold ved norske sykehjem – idealer og realiteter. *Vard i Norden* 2/2010. Publ. No. 96 Vol. 30 No. 2: 14-17.

Intrator, O., Castle, N.G., & Mor, V. 1999. Facility characteristics associated with hospitalization of nursing home residents: results of a national study. *Medical Care 37*(3): 228-237.

Intrator, O., Zinn, J., & Mor, V. 2004. Nursing home characteristics and potentially preventable hospitalizations of long-stay residents. *Journal of the American Geriatrics Society.* 52: 1730-1736.

Jablonski, R., Utz, S., Steeves, R. & Gray, D. 2007. Decisions about transfer from NH to emergency department. *Journal of Nursing Scholarship 39*(3): 266-272.

Jacobsen, F.F. 2004. Sykehjem – et hjem for deg og en arbeidsplass for meg? I Hugaas, J.V., Hummelvoll, J.K. & Solli, H.M. (eds.): *Helse og Helhet. Etiske og Tverrfaglige Perspektiver på Helsefaglig Teori og Praksis.* Oslo: UniPub Forlag.

Jacobsen, F.F. 2005. *Cultural Discontinuity as an Organizational Resource; Nursing in a Norwegian Nursing Home.* Research series No.3. NLA-Forlaget.

Jenkins, R. 1992. *Pierre Bourdieu.* Routledge, London.

Jensen, P.M., Fraser, F., Shankardass, K., Epstein, R.J.K. 2009. Are long-term residents referred appropriately to hospital emergency departments? *Can Fam Physician 5*(55): 500-505.

Kayser-Jones, J.S., Wiener, C.L. & Barbaccia, J.C. 1989. Factors contributing to the hospitalization of nursing home residents. *The Gerontologist 4,* Vol. 29: 502-510.

Kayser-Jones, J.S. 1990. *Old, Alone and Neglected. Care of the Aged in Scotland and the United States.* University of California Press.

Konetzka, R.T., Spector, W. & Schaffer, T. 2004. Effects of nursing home ownership type and resident payer source on hospitalization for suspected pneumonia. *Medical Care 10,* Vol. 42: 1001-1008.

Konetzka, R.T., Spector, W. & Limcangco, M.R: 2008. Reducing hospitalizations from long-term care settings. *Medical Care Research and Review 1,* Vol.65: 40-66.

Krüger, K., Jansen, K., Grimsmo, A., Eide, G.E., & Geitung, J.T. 2011. Hospital admissions from nursing homes: rates and reasons. *Nursing Research and Practice.* Vol. 2011: 1-6.

Laging, B., Ford, R., Bauer, M., & Nay, R. 2015. A meta-synthesis of factors influencing nursing home staff decisions to transfer residents to hospital. *Journal of Advanced Nursing* Oct *71*(10): 2224-2236.

Lamb, G., Tappen, R., Diaz, S., Herndon, L. & Ouslander, J. 2011. Avoidability of hospital transfers of NH residents: perspectives of frontline staff. *JAGS 59*(9): 1665-1672.

Larsen, K. & Adamsen, L. 2008. Emergence of Nordic nursing research: no position is an Island. *Scandinavian Journal of Caring Science* Dec *23*(4): 757-756

Lindgren, Gerd. 1992 *Doktorer Systrar och Flickor.* Carlssons Bokforlag. Stockholm.

Lloyd, L., Banerjee, A., Harrington, C., Jacobsen, F.F. & Szebehely, M. 2014. It is a scandal!: Comparing the causes and consequences of nursing home media scandals in five countries. *International Journal of Sociology and Social Policy*, Vol. 34 Iss: *1*(2): 2-18.

Loeb, M., Carusone, S.C., Goeree, R., Walter, S.D., Brazil, K., Krueger, P., Simor, A., Moss, L. & Marrie, T. 2006. Effect of a clinical pathway to reduce hospitalizations in nursing home residents with pneumonia–a randomized controlled trial. *JAMA*; 295: 2503-2510.

Lopez, R. 2009. Decision-making for acutely ill NH residents: nurses in the middle. *Journal of Advanced Nursing 65*(5): 1001-1009.

Lundgren, E. 2000. Homelike housing for elderly people? Materialized ideology. *Housing, Theory and Society 17*(3): 109-120.

Martin, P.Y. 2002. Sensations, bodies, and the 'spirit of a place': Aesthetics in residential organizations for the elderly. *Human Relations 55*(7): 861-885.

McCloskey, R.M. 2011. A qualitative study on the transfer of residents between a NH and an emergency department. *JAGS 59*: 717-724.

McCloskey, R. & Hoonaard, D.V.D. 2007. Nursing home residents in emergency departments: a Foulcauldian analysis. *Journal of Advanced Nursing 59*(2): 186-194.

McGregor, M., Pare, D., Wong, A., Cox, M.B., & Brasher, P. 2010. Correlates of a «do not hospitalize» designation: In a sample of frail nursing home residents in Vancouver. *Canadian Family Physician 56* (11): 1158-1164.

McGregor, M., Abu-Laban, R.B., Ronald, L.A., McGrail, K.M., Andrusiek, D., Baumbusch, J., Cox, M.B., Salomons, K., Schulzer, M., & Kuramoto, L. 2014. Nursing home characteristics associated with resident transfers to emergency departments. *Canadian Journal on Aging* Mar *33*(1): 38-48.

Miller, E.A. & Weissert, W.G. 2000. Predicting elderly people's risk for nursing home placement, hospitalization, functional impairment, and mortality: A synthesis. *Medical Care Research and Review* Vol. 57, No. 3: 359-397.

Ministry of Health and Care Services (HOD). 1989, *Forskrift for sykehjem og boform for heldøgns omsorg og pleie* [Regulations for nursing homes and facilities with 24 hour services]. Oslo.

Ministry of Health and Care Services (HOD). 2003. [1997] *Forskrift om kvalitet i pleie- og omsorgstjenestene for tjenesteyting,* [Regulations for quality in care services]. Oslo

Mitchell, G., Nicholson, C., McDonald, K. & Bucetti, A. 2011. Enhancing palliative care in rural Australia: the residential aged care setting. *Australian Journal of Primary Health* 17, 95-101.

Mor, V., Gruneir, A, Feng, Z., Grabowski, D.C., Intrator, O. & Zinn, J. 2010a. The effect of state policies on nursing home resident outcomes. *JAGS.* 59: 3-9.

Mor, V., Intrator, O., Feng, Z. & Grabowski, D.C. 2010b. The Revolving door of rehospitalization from skilled nursing facilities. *Health Affairs*, 29, No. 1: 57-64.

Murtaugh, C.M., & Freiman, M.P. 1995. Nursing home residents at risk of hospitalization and the characteristics of their hospital stays. *Gerontologist* Vol. 35. No 1: 35-43.

National Center for Health Statistics. 2013. Long Term Care Services in the United States: 2013 Overview. *National Health Care Statistics Report*, Number. 1.

NOU. 2004. *Norges Offentlige Utredninger: 18. Helhet og Plan i Sosial- og Helsetjenestene: Samhandling og Samordning i Kommunale Sosial- og Helsetjenester.* Statens Forvaltningstjeneste. Informasjonsforvaltning: Oslo.

Næss, A., & Vabø, M. 2012. Negotiating narratives of elderly care: The case of Pakistani migration to Norway. *Ageing International* Volume 39, Issue 1: 13-32.

Næss, A., Havig, A.K., & Vabø, M. 2013. Contested spaces — The perpetual quest for change in Norwegian nursing homes. In Hujala, A., Rissanen, S. & Vihma, S. (Eds.), *Designing Wellbeing in Elderly Care Homes* (pp. 68-83). Helsinki: Aalto University Publication Series, Crossover 2.

OECD. 2013. *Health at a Glance 2013: OECD Indicators*, OECD Publishing.

OIG. 2013. *Medicare Nursing Home Resident Hospitalization Rates Merit Additional Monitoring.* Office of Inspector General. Department of Health and Human Services. Rapport OEI-06-11-00040.

O'Malley, A.J., Caudry, D.J. & Grabowski, D.C. 2011. Predictors of nursing home residents' time to hospitalization. *Health Service Research* 46:1: 82-104.

O'Malley, A.J., Maracantonio, E.R., Murkofsky, R.L., Caudry, D.J., & Buchannan, J.l. 2007. Deriving a model of the necessity to hospitalize nursing home residents. *Research on Aging 29*: 606-625.

Otnes, B. 2015. Utviklingen i pleie- og omsorgstjenestene 1994-2013. *Tidsskrift for omsorgsforskning*, Vol.1, Nr. 1: 48-61.

Ouslander, J.G., Lamb, G., Perloe, M., Givens, J.H., Kluge, L., Rutland, T., Altherly, A., & Saliba, D. 2010. Potentially avoidable hospitalizations of nursing home residents: frequency, causes and costs. *Journal American Ger Society* 58: 627-635.

Ouslander, J.G. & Berenson, R.A. 2011. Reducing unnecessary hospitalizations of nursing home resident. *The New England Journal of Medicine* 365: 13: 1165-1167.

Pappas, G. & Hadden, W.C. 1997. Potentially avoidable hospitalizations: inequalities in rates between US socioeconomic groups. *Am J Public Health* 87: 811-816.

Parry, C., Coleman, E.A., Smith, J.D., Frank, J. & Kramer, A.M. 2003. The care transitions interventions: a patient-centered approach to ensuring effective transfers between sites of geriatric care. *Home Health Care Service Q*: 22: 1-16.

Petersen, K.A. 1993. *Den Praktiske Erkendelse. Forholdet Mellom Teori og Praksis i Sygeplejen og Sygeplejerskeuddannelsen*. Skrift-serie fra Danmarks Sygeplejerskehøjskole Nr 4, 1993. Aarhus Universitet.

Petersen, K.A. 1996. «Hvorfor Bourdieu?» *Fokus på Sygeplejen* 1996: 123-143, Munksgaard, København.

Petersen, K.A. 2004. Om teoriens rolle i profesjonspraktikker og uddannelser hertil. I Peteresen, K.A. (Ed.) *Praktikker i Erhverv og Uddannelse*. Frydenlund.

Petersen, K.A., & Callewaert, S. 2013. *Praxeologisk Sykeplejevidenskab: hvad er det? En Diskussion med det Subjektivistiske og det Objektivistiske Alternativ*. Bergen: Forlaget Hexis.

Phelan, E.A., Borson, S., Grothaus, L., Balch, S. & Larson, E.B. 2012. Association of incident dementia with hospitalizations. *Journal of American Medical Association*. Vol 307, No. 2: 165-172.

Phillips, J., Davidson, P., Jackson, M., Kristjanson, L., Daly, J. & Curran, J. 2006. Residential aged care: the last frontier for palliative care. *Journal of Advanced Nursing* 55(4): 416-424.

Prieur, Annick. 1993. Iscenesettelser av Kjønn; Transvestitter og Macho-menn i Mexico By. ISO Rapport Nr. 35. 1993. Institutt for sosiologi. Universitetet i Oslo.

Prieur, A. 2002. Objektivering og refleksivitet – om Pierre Bourdieus perspektiv på design og interview. I Hviid Jacobsen, M., Kristiansen, S. & Prieur, A. (Eds.) *Liv, Fortælling, Tekst. Streiftog i Kvalitativ Sociologi* (pp. 109-132). Aalborg Universitetsforlag.

Prieur, A. & Sestoft, C. 2006. *Pierre Bourdieu: En Introduksjon*. Hans Reitzels Forlag.

Read, S. 1999. Inappropriate admissions to hospital: the views of nursing and residential homes. *Nursing Standard 11*, Vol. 33: 32-35.

Rubenstein, L.Z., Josephson, K.R. & Osterweil, D. 1996. Falls and fall prevention in the nursing home. *Clinics in Geriatric Medicine* 12(4): 881-902.

Sandvoll, A.M. 2013. *Vi berre gjer det: beskrivingar av skjult pleiepraksis i sjukeheim.* Avhandling for graden philosophiae doctor (PhD). Universitetet i Bergen.

Schaffer, M.A. 2007. Ethical problems in end-of-life decisions for elderly Norwegians. *Nurs Ethics* 14: 242-257.

Selbæk, G., Kirkevold, Ø. & Engedal, K. 2007. The prevalence of psychiatric symptoms and behavioral disturbances and the use of psychotropic drugs in Norwegian nursing homes. *Int J Geriatr Psychiatry* 22: 843-849.

Shanley, C., Whitmore, E., Conforti, D., Masso, J., Jayasinghe, S. & Griffiths, R. 2011. Decisions about transferring NH residents to hospital: highlighting the roles of advance care planning and support from local hospital and community health services. *Journal of Clinical Nursing* 20(19-20): 2897-2906.

Shidler S. 1998. A systemic perspective of life-prolonging treatment decision-making. *Qualitative Health Research* 8(2): 254-269.

SINTEF. 2009. *Eldreomsorgen i Norge: Helt utilstrekkelig – eller best i verden.* Sintef helsetjenesteforskning 2009.

Slagsvold, B. 1986. *Sykehjemmet – et Sosialt System.* NGI-rapport 3/86, Oslo.

Spector, W., Shaffer, T., Potter, D.E.B., Correa-de-Araujo, R. & Limcango, M.R. 2007. Risk factors associated with the occurrence of fractures in U.S. nursing homes: resident and facility characteristics and prescription medications. *Journal of the American Geriatrics Society.* 55: 327-333.

SSB. 2010. *Individbasert statistikk for pleie- og omsorgstjenesten i kommunene (IPLOS),* Statistisk sentralbyrå Rapporter 50/2010.

Steen, K., Mjeldheim, M., & Hunskår, S. 2009. Legevakt for alders- og sykehjemmene. *Tidsskrift for Den norske legeforening.* Nr. 21: 129: 2223-2225.

Stephens, C.E., Newcomer, R., Blegen, M., Miller, B. & Harrington, C. 2011. Emergency department use by nursing home residents: effect of severity of cognitive impairment. *Gerontologist* Jun 52(3): 383-393.

Stortingsmelding nr. 25 (2005-2006). 2006. *Mestring, muligheter og mening.* Helse- og omsorgsdepartementet, Oslo.

Stortingsmelding nr. 26 (2014-2015). 2015. *Fremtidens primærhelsetjeneste – nærhet og omsorg.* Helse- og omsorgsdepartementet, Oslo.

Stortingsmelding nr. 47 (2008-2009). 2009. *Samhandlingsreformen. Rett behandling – på rett sted – til rett tid.* Helse- og omsorgsdepartementet, Oslo.

Stortingsmelding nr. 50 (1996-1997). 1997. *Handlingsplan for eldreomsorgen – trygghet – respekt – kvalitet.* Helse- og omsorgsdepartementet, Oslo.

Terrell, K.M. & Miller, D.K. 2006. Challenges in transitional care between NHs and emergency departments. *Journal of the American Medical Directors Association* 7(8): 499-505.

Vabø, M., Christensen, K., Trætteberg, H.D., & Jacobsen, F.F. 2013. Marketization in Norwegian eldercare. Preconditions, trends and resistance. In Meagher, G. & Szebehely, M. (Eds.), *Marketisation in Nordic Eldercare: Legislation, Oversight, Extent and Consequences* (pp. 163-202). Stockholm University: Department of Social Work.

Vike, H. 2003. Byråkratiske utopier. Om etableringen av orden i offentlig forvaltning. *Norsk Antropologisk Tidsskrift 2-3*. Vol. 14: 122-136.

Vossius, C.E., Ydstebø, A.E., Testad, I., & Lurås, H. 2013. Referrals from nursing home to hospitals: Reasons, appropriateness and costs. Scandinavian Journal of Public Health. 41: 366-373.

Walker, J.D., Teare, G.F., Hogan, D.B., Lewis, S. & Maxwell, C.J. 2009. Identifying potentially avoidable hospital admissions from Canadian long-term care facilities. *Med Care* 47: 250-254.

Weech-Maldonado, R., Meret-Hanke, L., Neff, M.C., & Mor, V. 2004. Nurse staffing patterns and quality of care in nursing homes. *Health Care Management Review*. 29: 107-116.

Wennberg, J, Barnes, B, & Zubkoff, M. 1982. Professional uncertainty and the problem of supplier-induced demand. *Social Science and Medicine* 1982; *16*(7): 811-824.

Wærness, K. 1984. The rationality of caring. *Economic and Industrial Democracy 5*(2): 185-211.

Zimmerman, S., Gruber-Baldini, A.L., Hebel, J.R., Sloane, P.D. & Magaziner, J. 2002. Nursing home facility risk factors for infection and hospitalization: importance of registered nurse turnover, administration, and social factors. *Journal of the American Geriatrics Society* 50: 1987-1995.

Ågotnes, G. 2005. *To be or not to be: Om strategier for overlevelse, maktkamp og vennskap i et kostskolehus.* Masteroppgave institutt for sosialantropologi, Universitetet i Bergen.

Ågotnes, G., Jacobsen, F.F., Harrington, C. & Pettersen, K.A. 2015. A critical review of research on hospitalization from nursing homes; What is missing? Ageing International. Vol 41. Issue 1: 3-16

www.ingramcontent.com/pod-product-compliance
Lightning Source LLC
Chambersburg PA
CBHW080252030726

47593CB00009B/2461